Fast Facts for CAREER SUCCESS IN NURSING: *Making the Most of Mentoring in a Nutshell,* Vance

Fast Facts for DEVELOPING A NURSING ACADEMIC PORTFOLIO: *What You Really Need to Know in a Nutshell,* Wittmann-Price

Fast Facts for the CLASSROOM NURSING INSTRUCTOR: *Classroom Teaching in a Nutshell,* Yoder-Wise, Kowalski

Forthcoming FAST FACTS Books

Fast Facts for the MEDICAL–SURGICAL NURSE: *Clinical Orientation in a Nutshell,* Ciocco

Fast Facts for the OPERATING ROOM NURSE: *An Orientation and Care Guide in a Nutshell,* Criscitelli

Fast Facts for the LONG-TERM CARE NURSE: *A Guide for Nurses in Nursing Homes and Assisted Living Settings,* Eliopoulos

Fast Facts for the ONCOLOGY NURSE: *Oncology Nursing Orientation in a Nutshell,* Lucas

Fast Facts for the TRIAGE NURSE: *An Orientation and Care Guide in a Nutshell,* Montejano, Grossman

Fast Facts for the PEDIATRIC NURSE: *An Orientation Guide in a Nutshell,* Rupert, Young

Visit www.springerpub.com to order.

FAST FACTS ON ADOLESCENT HEALTH FOR NURSING AND HEALTH PROFESSIONALS

Judith Wheaton Herrman, PhD, RN, ANEF, has been a pediatric nurse for over 30 years, working as a staff nurse, nurse manager, nurse educator, researcher, and advocate. Her programs of research focus on adolescent health and decision-making, teens having a voice in their health care and decisions, sexual development, teen pregnancy prevention, and addressing teen dating violence. In this role, she has been fascinated by teen brain development and its impact on behavior and health. Her interface with teens, nursing students, community resources, health care agencies, adolescent-focused advocates and professionals, and other consumers positions her as a leader in adolescent nursing. She is currently a professor at the School of Nursing, University of Delaware, Newark, Delaware. Dr. Herrman is the author of numerous scholarly publications and research grants, and is a popular and highly regarded speaker and lecturer on many topics related to teen health and education across the life span. She is also the recipient of many distinguished nursing awards and honors, including being a Fellow in the American Academy of Nursing Education.

FAST FACTS ON ADOLESCENT HEALTH FOR NURSING AND HEALTH PROFESSIONALS

A Care Guide in a Nutshell

Judith Wheaton Herrman, PhD, RN, ANEF

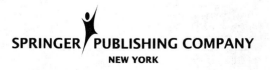

SPRINGER PUBLISHING COMPANY
NEW YORK

Springer Publishing Company, LLC
11 West 42nd Street
New York, NY 10036
www.springerpub.com

Acquisitions Editor: *Elizabeth Nieginski*
Composition: S4Carlisle Publishing Services

ISBN: 978-0-8261-7145-0
e-book ISBN: 978-0-8261-7146-7

14 15 16 / 5 4 3 2 1

The author and the publisher of this Work have made every effort to use sources believed to be reliable to provide information that is accurate and compatible with the standards generally accepted at the time of publication. Because medical science is continually advancing, our knowledge base continues to expand. Therefore, as new information becomes available, changes in procedures become necessary. We recommend that the reader always consult current research and specific institutional policies before performing any clinical procedure. The author and publisher shall not be liable for any special, consequential, or exemplary damages resulting, in whole or in part, from the readers' use of, or reliance on, the information contained in this book. The publisher has no responsibility for the persistence or accuracy of URLs for external or third-party Internet websites referred to in this publication and does not guarantee that any content on such websites is, or will remain, accurate or appropriate.

Library of Congress Cataloging-in-Publication Data

Herrman, Judith W., author.
  Fast facts on adolescent health for nursing and health professionals : a care guide in a nutshell / Judith Wheaton Herrman.
    p. ; cm. — (Fast facts)
  Includes bibliographical references and index.
  ISBN-13: 978-0-8261-7145-0
  ISBN-10: 0-8261-7145-1
  ISBN-13: 978-0-8261-7146-7 (e-book)
  I. Title. II. Series: Fast facts (Springer Publishing Company)
  [DNLM: 1. Pediatric Nursing—methods. 2. Adolescent Behavior. 3. Adolescent Medicine—methods. 4. Adolescent Psychology. 5. Attitude of Health Personnel. WY 159]
  RJ550
  616.00835—dc23
                            2014004347

Printed in the United States of America by Gasch Printing.

This book, in which I share my thoughts on adolescent health, is dedicated to my parents (who knew me as an adolescent), to my husband (who did not but whose wisdom about life and teens continues to inspire me), to my three sons and their wives (who taught me to love adolescents and adolescence), and to my three grandchildren (who are now infants), who will provide me with ongoing purpose, dedication to and interest in the adolescent years.

Contents

x

CONTENTS

Part III: Aspects of Caring for the Adolescent With Illness and Complex Health Issues

Preface

As Margaret Mead stated, "the solution to adult problems tomorrow depends in large measure upon the way our children grow up today. There is no greater insight into the future than recognizing that, when we save our children, we save ourselves."

I believe this is especially true of adolescents, who establish health beliefs and patterns, learn decision-making, and become the productive and active adults of tomorrow. Adults interacting with teens, whether in their personal or professional lives, know the rewards, challenges, and sometimes the mysteries of these experiences. This book is designed to assist health care professionals to understand and to be successful in these interactions, to have positive impacts on teens, and to advocate effectively for youth. Adolescent development, factors affecting teen health, suggestions for working and communicating with teens, and issues impacting adolescents in six holistic health domains are addressed. Selected issues facing teens with acute and chronic illness, matters associated with teens and technology, legal and ethical issues, and the marginalization of youth challenge readers to ponder their perceptions about adolescents. This book is unique in its concise presentation, comprehensive nature, easy-to-reference information, and positive approach to the teen years. Chapter objectives, informative lists and tables, key facts, synthesis of major issues, and references for future study make this book an important resource for health care professionals who are working with teens and are blessed with teens in their lives!

Judith Wheaton Herrman

Overview of Adolescence

The Wonderful Teen

Many of us find that the time we spend with teens—in our work, home, or community—is some of the most rewarding, albeit challenging, of our lives. Observing the teen mind work, process, and come up with unique conclusions is a very special part of what we do. Other times we may find teens defiant, lacking perspective, or just simply frustrating. Our responses to adolescents may depend upon the individual teen, our thoughts and moods, our own teen experience, and our expectations of behavior and how today's youth conforms. Environmental and social factors, such as culture, community norms, poverty, current events, family and family structure, and ongoing stressors may impact teens' behaviors and our interactions with them. Rather than clutching on to the media's depictions of "teens gone wild" or the escapades of teens who refrain from considering negative consequences, we should consider the positive aspects of the teen years. Teens are an important and vital age group in our society. They play a critical role as they become the workforce, inventors, and decision-makers of tomorrow.

In this chapter, you will learn to:

1. Define the years associated with adolescence
2. Discuss the importance of a positive, partnership approach when working with teens
3. Use the six health domains approach to holistically view teens
4. Identify key focused interventions based upon learned concepts

Some perspectives on teens as presented in this text:

- We focus on the positive nature of adolescents as they grow and develop.
- We consider interactions with teens as valuable partnerships rather than "us-against-them" relationships.
- Teen development is an ongoing process of engagement with friends, adults, and institutions, and teens' own perspectives that frame their individual responses, thoughts, and actions.
- We do not engage in "ephebephobia," or the irrational fear of adolescence. Instead, we believe that teens are exciting, interesting, and always changing.
- Developmental theory tells us that as humans mature, sensitive periods emerge during which skills and milestones are attained. Just as we would not expect an infant to walk prior to the appropriate time during development, teens accomplish age-related tasks at logical and sequential critical periods in their development.
- We can use information on teens and development to teach and provide anticipatory guidance for teens, families, and others to foster healthy youth and young adults.
- We can better establish relationships with teens armed with knowledge about teen growth and development, the potential idiosyncrasies of the teen years, and ways adults can foster development and preserve the individuality and enthusiasm of each teen.

DEFINING ADOLESCENCE

Everyone has his or her own thoughts on the years beginning and ending the adolescent period. Some see adolescence as a transition period where individuals are not quite children but also not yet adults. The years that encompass the period of adolescence are largely socially constructed and dependent upon the norms, beliefs, and behaviors of society.

Definitions of the teen years may be based on economic factors, biological characteristics, and the experiences inherent of the time period. Our personal experiences, the demands of society, the people with whom we interact, and changing conceptualizations of age-appropriate behaviors all impact our definitions.

The current accepted definition of adolescence describes the second decade of life, usually ages 10 to 24 years. The lower age of adolescence may vary based on a variety of factors, most importantly the onset of puberty. This age has lowered in recent years; in the 1900s, puberty occurred around 16 years of age and today it occurs around age 10, potentially due to advances in nutrition, health, and health care.

The early years of adolescence, called the "tween years," provide a preface for adolescence. The term "teenagers" was introduced in the post–World War II marketing world. Adolescent wage earners, previously integral to supporting the family economy as their earnings supplemented the family income, now became a group with discretionary income. They were able to buy record albums, clothes, drinks at the soda shop, and gas for their cars, and were able to afford other things, boosting the economy. Thus, the new age cohort of teenagers was born out of social and economic conditions.

Much more difficult to identify in America is when adolescence ends. The age at which teens bear children, establish independence from parents, begin careers, and enter into adult lives may also be influenced by schooling, the presence of adult supports and role models, and the personal characteristics of the individual.

As we will discover, stages of adolescent brain development may also inform this discussion. Teens who do not attend secondary education, begin childbearing early, and establish young-adult lifestyles in the late teens become young adults. Others who continue schooling well into their 20s may continue their years of dependency, both financially and otherwise, and be considered adolescents for longer periods. The end of adolescence, therefore, may be considered at ages 18, 22, 25, or older based on the individual. Authors now discuss the period of the "emerging adult" to characterize this late adolescence period.

We should consider that while we may generalize the behaviors of teens based on their chronological age, each is an individual with unique abilities, gifts, and strengths. Each teen differs from his or her peers based on physiological, genetic, environmental, experiential, and other factors. Although this book discusses commonalities among teens and their stage of development, we also appreciate the uniqueness of each teen we work with and the need to individualize our thoughts and actions to ensure personalized care.

FAST FACTS in a NUTSHELL

The years accepted as adolescence are shaped by social norms. The accepted years denoting adolescence today include ages 10 to 24 years.

THE VALUE OF TEENS IN OUR WORLD

Children were not always valued by society as they are today. Significant rates of infant and child mortality, the economic burden of children, conflicting views of gender, and social views of the developing child all influenced a rather negative view of children. The phrase "children are to be seen and not heard" reinforced the role of children in the family and the way children were treated. Adolescence, then, was viewed as a transition period—the time between this era of little value and when adults, who really count, emerge. We now see adolescence differently, yet sometimes continue to devalue the adolescent years. At times we treat teens as emerging adults and tolerate them until they "grow out" of their difficult ways. Instead, perhaps our thoughts about teens should consider that we were all teens once, and that we confronted difficult times and issues, experienced newness and excitement as only teens can, and learned to become adults. The experiences of our teen years helped shape who we are today. Likewise, our interactions with teens have long-lasting impact on each young person with whom we work and how he or she grows and develops. Dealing with teens with humility is how adults can approach teens on a healthy and meaningful level—our role is to help shape them to be the best adults they can be. Interventions that may foster this development are found throughout this book. Through focused interventions in our work as nurses or other health care providers with youth, we emphasize the uniqueness of adolescents and the emphasis on developmentally appropriate care. Assessment of developmental abilities along with chronological age ensures developmentally appropriate care. We must do this not *for* teens, but *with* teens. We need their thoughts, opinions, and perspectives to assist us to help them grow!

Some thoughts on working with teens:

- Teens have engaged in conflict and discord with adults down through the ages. As quoted by Socrates in the 5th century BCE: "Our youth now love luxury. They have bad manners...contempt for authority...they show disrespect for their elders...favor chatter in place of exercise...they contradict their parents, gobble up food, and tyrannize their teachers."
- This discord may allow teens to separate themselves from their adult caregivers, establish personal and individual identities, and seek out new thoughts and ideas about the changing world.
- Teens' levels of energy, attraction to risk behaviors, and lack of appreciation of hindrances may be seen as impulsive, risk laden, and lacking forethought. Adults may avoid risk, focus on negative consequences, and fear change, which hinder progress and reinforce stagnation. In converse, teen behaviors allow for creativity, discovery, and excitement.

- Adults need to embrace teens and their energy, allowing teens to grow and flourish within safe and healthy parameters.

We discuss teen behaviors from the perspective of realistic consequences, rationales for teen actions, and how we may foster healthy decision-making and healthy behavior. It is in discovering the confines of the parameters of behavior that adults and teens may clash, requiring empathy, understanding, and patience.

HEALTH DOMAINS IN VIEWING TEENS

To ensure that this text provides a comprehensive view of teens, their health, and health care implications, young people are viewed from health domains that are equally important when viewing the holistic individual. These domains are noted in Table 1.1.

Viewing each domain independently allows us to appreciate the importance of each sector and how alterations in each may impact the individual. Further exploration of how these discriminant elements within the larger constellation of youth behavior enables us to view the whole person, the impact of the domains on each other, and how to assist teens as they progress through their adolescent years.

TABLE 1.1 The Health Domains

Physical

Intellectual

Emotional

Spiritual

Sexual

Relational

- Consider developmental and chronological age when assessing individual teens.
- Provide unconditional support of teens and differentiate the person, and your esteem for him or her, from the behavior and its ramifications.
- Remember your own teen years as you continue to explore teens' health needs, priorities, and concerns.
- Assist teens in understanding, but not being stifled by, the potential consequences of actions.
- Although commonalities exist, remember that each teen remains a unique individual.
- Focus on the positive energy of teens rather than on the more negative or sensationalized images of today's teens.
- Partnering with teens, seeking their thoughts and opinions, and validating teens as valuable, important members of society are critical as we assist teens to grow and flourish.

SUGGESTED READING

Arnett, J. J. (2010). Oh grow up! Generational grumbling and the new life state of emerging adulthood. *Perspectives on Psychological Science, 5*(1), 89–92.

Blakemore, S. J., & Choudhury, S. (2006). Development of the adolescent brain: Implications for executive function and social cognition. *Journal of Child Psychology and Psychiatry, 47*(3/4), 296–312.

Bray, D. (2011). *Growing great girls: A life skills curriculum for girls.* Wilmington, DE: DGI.

McNeely, C., & Blanchard, J. (2009). *The teen years explained: A guide to healthy adolescent development.* Baltimore, MD: Johns Hopkins Bloomburg School of Public Health.

Steinberg, L. (2008). *Adolescence.* New York, NY: McGraw-Hill.

SUGGESTED WEBSITES

Kids Health.Org
www.kidshealth.org/teen

Healthy Teen Network
www.healthyteennetwork.org

Advocates for Youth
www.advocatesforyouth.org

The Youth Activism Project
www.youthactivism.org

The Search Institute
www.search-institute.org

CityMatch
www.citymatch.org

Child Trends
www.childtrends.org

The National Campaign to Prevent Teen and Unplanned Pregnancy
www.nationalcampaign.org

Johns Hopkins School of Public Health
www.jhsph.edu

Healthy People
www.healthypeople.gov

Society for Adolescent Medicine and Health
www.adolescenthealth.org

University of Minnesota Extension
http://www1.extension.umn.edu/family/cyfc/our-services

The Innovation Center
www.theinnovationcenter.org

2

The Teen Brain

Teens think differently than adults. Advanced diagnostics can now pinpoint the parts of the brain that are responsible for different functions, the response of the brain to stimuli, and the impact of different environmental, health, and experiential factors on the ability to respond and act. Scientists are able to analyze brain function more precisely than ever before, leading to ongoing discoveries about the development of the teen brain and the impact of maturation on decision-making and behavior.

In this chapter, you will learn to:

1. Describe the changes in the brain as teens develop and mature
2. Discuss how brain development impacts how teens interpret risks and rewards
3. Describe the role of maturation in the development of empathy and emotional interpretation
4. Identify key focused interventions based upon learned concepts

Early research indicated that the brain largely developed during the early years of life and the subsequent years yielded an ongoing, but less impressive, level of growth. Scientists now know that the teen years are a time of vast growth and development, and that monumental changes occur during this time that may provide insights into some teen behavior. Just knowing about these changes and the level of brain growth during the teen years can guide us toward a better understanding of the behaviors of this unique age group.

THE THREE PROCESSES OF BRAIN DEVELOPMENT

The development of the teen brain occurs in a predictable pattern throughout the teen years, beginning in the back of the brain and progressing forward. It is not known exactly at which ages this brain development begins and ends, but knowledge of these processes helps us understand some aspects of teen behavior characteristic of early, middle, and late adolescence. For our purposes, these characteristic time frames include:

- Early teen years: 10 to 13 years of age
- Middle teen years: 14 to 17 years of age
- Late teen years: 18 to 24 years of age

FAST FACTS in a NUTSHELL

It is during these time frames that three main processes of brain development take place: proliferation, pruning, and myelinization.

Proliferation

- Proliferation is the rapid growth in the number of neurons in the brain.
- Neurons are the basic unit of function in the brain and are responsible for transmission of impulses that bring

information from sensory cells to the brain for interpretation and for return of the impulses to effector, or
response, cells to act.
- Proliferation peaks in early adolescence, around
  11 years in girls and 12½ years in boys.
- It is often thought that the "glazed look" in the eyes
  of "tweens" may be attributed to this rapid accumu-
  lation of nerve cells within the brain. As the brain
  gets "bushier," the young teen brain may experience
  "white noise" or interference as it negotiates problems
  and tries to sift through large amounts of data in the
  growing brain.

Pruning

- Pruning describes a less known or understood process
  in reaction to the overproduction of nerve cells during
  proliferation.
- Just like an overcrowded dresser drawer in your home
  that finally demands "decluttering," pruning assists
  the brain to clean out nerve cells by cutting away those
  cells that are less used.
- This "use-it-or-lose-it" mechanism of pruning, perhaps the greatest discovery associated with MRI brain
  research, delineates that those cells that are used are
  strengthened, allowing for stronger and faster connections of nerve transmission, while those that are less
  used atrophy and die away.
- Research is cautious about the ability to "selectively
  prune" the "hardwiring of the brain" in our teens, but
  this does inform our need to expose teens to varied and
  interesting stimuli, guide youth development, provide
  mentoring as teens confront new and different situations, and allow some degree of independence as teens
  make choices and seek out new experiences.
- Pruning, and the brain energy devoted to this process,
  may require the provision of additional time and opportunities for decision-making in order for teens to
  handle conflicts or decisions.

- It is believed that this pruning phase begins in the middle teen years and continues well into the 20s, and is impacted by experience, genetics, hormones, nutrition, substance use, and environmental factors.

Myelinization

- The third process is myelinization, or the covering of neurons with a protective coating.
- Much like the plastic coating of insulation on a copper wire contains the energy and makes electrical conduction more efficient, the fatty myelin layer insulates each nerve cell and increases the speed and efficiency of nerve impulse transmission.
- Myelinization also allows the brain to attend to multiple stimuli and to do so simultaneously.
- Myelination is thought to slow the learning process and make it more difficult to heal when injured. This is why these processes are hindered in adults who have largely myelinated neurons.

Many believe that the myelinization process alone may explain the superior ability of adults to appreciate the consequences of behavior more than teens. For example, it was previously considered that teen drivers' apparent reluctance to brake at a stop sign until the last minute was due to the faster reaction time inherent in a younger age. In contrast, newer research tells us that teens are slower to process incoming stimuli due to these unmyelinated cells, leading teens to react differently than adults and appear more impulsive or sudden in their actions. Adults, with greater percentages of myelinated cells, see the threat and immediately begin to process the potential positive and negative consequences of the situation and possible action alternatives. This process impacts teen behaviors as they propose to participate in an activity. While adults are considering the potential outcomes, teens are still focusing on the fun, stimulating, and novel aspects of the activity.

The processes of proliferation, pruning, and myelin-ization may explain teen thinking and behavior as the brain develops. These three processes begin in the back of the brain and progress to the front of the brain throughout adolescence. Knowledge about teen brain development is critical when working with youth.

BACK-TO-FRONT PROGRESSION

Understanding the maturation of each brain area enables us to better understand the accomplishment of developmental tasks and behaviors at certain ages during the teen years.

Back of the Brain

- Early in the teen years (ages 11 to 13), the back of the brain, including the amygdala and cerebellum, matures.
- The amygdala, often referred to as the "beast within us," generates our primitive emotional instincts and primal responses to stimuli, yielding such reactions as anger, rage, and fear.
- Early in the adolescent period, teens' reactions to dis-tressing situations may result from these primitive responses without the benefit of balance of the cogni-tive controls that later develop in the front of the brain.
- The developing amygdala may generate responses pre-viously thought of as "raging hormones," but instead, may be manifestations of early attempts to cope with conflict.
- The amygdala also allows for the cultivation of spirit, enthusiasm, and creativity without the constraints of self-consciousness, negative thoughts, or potential repercussions.

- The cerebellum, in addition to being responsible for fine and gross motor activities, the senses, physical co-ordination, and early thought processes, is the region of the brain largely influencing the connection of mind and body experiences.
- Newer research elaborates on the assets of exercise on brain development, the role of physical movement in problem solving, and the importance of activity on learning.
- Early skills in decision-making and mental planning originate from this region of the brain.

Middle Brain

- One of the parts of the middle brain is the basal ganglia. It is known as the "administrative assistant" of the brain, where skills in priority setting, organization, and assuming responsibility develop.
- Maturation of the middle brain allows teens to begin to understand how to manage a project. We often expect teens to embrace new projects in the same manner that adults would confront these tasks. In contrast, the developing teen brain warrants progressive independence as teens tackle complex projects. This ability to sequentially plan, see the order of a project, and anticipate next steps is a critical component of adolescent learning.

Front of the Brain

- Perhaps the most classic "discovery" about the brain occurred with the isolation and understanding of the function of the prefrontal cortex (PFC) in the front of the brain.
- Although the brain injury of a railroad worker in the mid-1800s alerted scientists to the important role of the front of the brain, it was not until later that scientists began to understand how the PFC works and why its function is critical in human behavior.

Phineas Gage was a railroad worker injured when a large rod pierced through his cheek and out the top of his head. Miraculously, predating anesthesia or antibiotics, Phineas lived for several more years after his injury, but with a total change in disposition. This previously kind, hard-working, and sincere man became belligerent, prone to fighting, and angry. What Phineas was missing, subsequent to his injury, was the part of the brain responsible for the "sober second thought."

- The PFC allows us to consider consequences, plan in our mental workspace, inhibit impulses, delay gratification, weigh the benefits and rewards of our actions, empathize with others, and "do the right thing."

We all can relate to times when we were tempted to do something impulsive. We considered our options, resisted temptation, and decided that it wasn't worth the effort to encounter the potential consequences. These executive functions collect information, organize thoughts, and anticipate differences between what will happen and what might happen. We also know that back in our teen years, much like the young people of today, we encountered situations in which we acted without using the filtering and decision-making mechanism developed within our PFC. By providing the cognitive controls over acts, the PFC functions to regulate behavior, consider ramifications, and develop mature responses to others in our world. Without a mature PFC, teens are unable to evaluate the ramifications of risk behavior or weigh their options in acting on impulses.

TEEN BEHAVIOR: RISKS AND REWARDS

Risks

One variable leading to risky behavior in teens is their natural tendency for sensation seeking. Some of this "appetite for thrills" is related to a neurotransmitter in the brain called do-pamine. Dopamine allows neurotransmissions to be carried from cell to cell and appears to be the origin of the teen brain's physiological desire for novel, risky, and intense stimuli.

- It is believed that teens seek out sensational experiences, risk behaviors, or events with a "bigger rush" to attain increasingly higher levels of pleasure and to satisfy their growing yearning for excitement.
- Sensation seeking is a natural, evolutionary trait in order to ensure that we seek out new experiences and discover and embrace opportunity, while promoting inventiveness and creativity.

FAST FACTS in a NUTSHELL

New attention is being devoted to one teen risk behavior—gambling. About 60% to 80% of teens reported gambling activity in the past year. Most are considered social or recreational gamblers, but 10% to 15% of those who gamble are thought to be at risk for a gambling problem and 3% to 8% are labeled pathologic gamblers. The Internet and social media have changed the way gambling appears on the landscape of teen behavior.

- Although all teens may be considered "at risk" for sensation-seeking behaviors, some are considered more vulnerable to dangerous behaviors. It is believed that once a teen participates in a risky behavior it is very easy to engage in further behaviors, as if participation in one imprudent act may lower the threshold for other risky behaviors.
- The highest levels of dopamine are found in 11- to 18-year-old youth. Essentially, teens are more dopamine dependent than adults and also need more intense stimuli to create pleasurable responses. We all know of teens who claim to be bored with day-to-day activities, which never seem to be enough to stimulate a teen.

TABLE 2.1 Healthy Strategies to Enhance Dopamine	
Engage in physical activity	Engage in acts of kindness
Savor feelings of accomplishment	Enjoy falling in love
Use humor	Embrace a sense of uniqueness
Seek positive interactions	Savor intense emotions

We may also remember the excitement of holidays as a child, when our dopamine levels surged. As we matured, these levels of dopamine declined and accounted for adult levels of contentment with less excitement.

- We know that teens may seek high-risk behaviors, with potential negative impacts, to feed this need for dopamine. Their lack of cognitive controls, poor impulse control, perceptions of peer pressure, and less developed sense of empathy may lead to health and safety issues.

- If teens are unable to get their "dopamine rush" in healthy ways, they may resort to unhealthy means to get these feelings. Table 2.1 includes healthy ways to enhance dopamine levels.

The PFC provides the cognitive controls for impulsive, pleasure-seeking actions or the tendency toward "if it feels good, do it." The ability to delay gratification, difficult for many in today's society, and to self-regulate impulses may be the product of the maturing PFC. "The temporal gap," or the delay of cognitive controls to completely appraise a situation prior to engaging in a behavior that meets pleasure-seeking needs, may serve to enhance teens' participation in high-risk behaviors.

The Role of Serotonin

Serotonin is the balancing neurotransmitter that levels out surges in dopamine and suppresses the urge for sensation seeking. Known to be a mood stabilizer, serotonin decreases the acute "appetite for thrills" and allows for feelings of contentment and satisfaction.

- Teens actually have lower levels of serotonin than adults, although for most teens this is not a significant problem. It may explain the negative affect and sullenness noted in some teens.
- As we age, our serotonin levels enable us to be content with less exciting stimuli and to have less of a need for risk-taking behavior.
- On the downside, as we get older we take fewer risks, may be less creative, oppose change, and pursue more safe, known behaviors rather than seeking new and different adventures. The converse is an exciting attribute of the teen years in which teens take risks, exude enthusiasm, and strive for different and unique experiences.

Rewards

- The teen brain, and resulting teen behavior, is wired to respond to rewards more than costs or negative consequences.
- The maturing nucleus accumbens is able to discern rewards, and dopamine is released upon the reward experience. Teens seek out rewarding experiences to have this dopamine "high," making them more sensitive to rewards.
- Teens often engage in high-excitement, low-effort activities, such as video games, in order to feel these positive reward effects during their everyday lives.
- Punishment, or the threat of consequences, does not seem to have the same impact on withholding dopamine or changing the way teens consider engagement in a behavior or decision-making.

Perhaps we remember interventions and curricula that used negative consequences to foster avoidance of high-risk behaviors. Showing pictures of advanced stages of sexually transmitted diseases, black lungs from cigarette smoking, or eggs frying in a pan to resemble brains after drug use all appeared to be convincing ways to reinforce avoiding high-risk behaviors. However, newer research dictates that teens do not reason abstractly, cannot make the connections that these negative consequences may represent their personal realities, and lack the future orientation to make sense of these strategies. Teens respond more to rewards-based interventions focusing on the positive aspects of avoiding such behaviors. The benefits of not smoking to play sports is both immediately relevant and attends to the rewards circuits of remaining smoke free, rather than traditional emphasis on long-term smoking leading to chronic respiratory disease, cancer, and heart disease. The ability to delay rewards and gratification, anticipate long-term impacts, and develop patience is believed to be closely linked with the maturing teen brain. Teens' increasing abilities to choose between positive and negative consequences, reason abstractly, and develop a future orientation impact how teens view their health and behaviors.

EMPATHY AND EMOTIONS

Another aspect of teen brain maturation is that of the development of empathy and emotional interpretation.

- The portion of the brain believed to be responsible for empathy, the cingulate gyrus, is found in the limbic area, or the emotional control center, of the brain. This area, as do all the parts of the brain, undergoes proliferation, pruning, and myelinization throughout the teen years.
- Newer research indicates that empathy forms earlier in girls than in boys and is predicated on puberty, timing of maturation, gender expectations, and opportunity to practice skills.
- Current research on the means to foster empathy in teens as ways to avoid risk behavior, develop a conscience, and appreciate social justice will continue to inform what we know about empathy and teen brain development.

The Role of Emotional Interpretation

Emotional interpretation, or the ability of the teen to correctly "read" the emotions of others, may be a portion of empathy development as teens gain insight into the thoughts and emotions of others. Adults use portions of the PFC to make cognitive decisions about the facial expressions of another individual and interpret the emotion associated with expressions, gestures, or body language. Teens use more posterior, less mature regions of their brain to make these interpretations.

Research done with "reading" of emotions based on pictures of eyes and facial expressions noted that teens are less able than adults to validly identify the facial expressions or emotions of others. We have all heard a teen say "that teacher hates me." The egocentricity of the teen years, wherein teens believe they must be at the root of the emotions of others, and teens' inability to accurately interpret these emotions, may lead teens to make suppositions about the thoughts of others. Teens essentially feel before they interpret and may have difficulty engaging in conversations about emotions. Accurate interpretation of emotions is important, as indicated in Table 2.2.

This summary of adolescent brain development, and its implications, provides the foundation for interventions

---

TABLE 2.2 Interpretation of Emotions

Emotional interpretation is important in:

Forming relationships	Avoiding fighting
Developing timing of discussions and behaviors	Emotional appraisal of situations
Communicating based on emotions	Reasoning based on emotional cues
Developing an intuitive sense or "gut feeling"	Developing empathy

designed to foster health and well-being. The investigation and clarification of teen brain maturation is not meant to be an excuse for bad behavior, nor does it wholly define teen behavior. Other influences such as the environment, genetics, and experiences work to shape the adults we become. Instead, it is meant to ensure that health care providers provide developmentally appropriate adolescent care based on current knowledge.

FOCUSED INTERVENTIONS

- Provide step-wise instructions at increasing levels of complexity as teens mature. Allow them to feel the positives of accomplishments while always learning and growing.
- Help teens identify the potential short- and long-term impacts of behavior, both the positive and the negative, and allow teens to develop decision-making skills with the support of a caring adult.
- Provide positive ways to experience novel and sensation-seeking behaviors inherent in the teen years and the supervision needed when impulses to seek out more risky behaviors emerge.
- Teach teens about emotional communication, empathy, and expression of emotions. Use art, drama, journaling, and other means to reach teens and help them connect with others.
- Help teens develop a "gut" reaction to potentially harmful situations based on experience, adult guidance, and increasing wisdom inherent in maturation.
- Assist parents in appreciating their powerful role in teens' lives by role modeling, supervision, monitoring, and education. For families with limited parental resources or abilities, refer the teen or family to support systems to ensure adequate guidance of teens through these growing years.

SUGGESTED READING

Blakemore, S. J., & Choudhury, S. (2006). Development of the adolescent brain: Implications for executive function and social cognition. *Journal of Child Psychology and Psychiatry, 47*(3/4), 296–312.

DeLisi, M., Wright, J. P., Vaughn, M. G., & Beaver, K. M. (2010). Nature and nurture by definition means both: A response to males. *Journal of Adolescent Research, 25*(1), 24–30.

Feinstein, S. (2007). *Teaching the at-risk teenage brain.* Lanham, MD: Rowman & Littlefield.

Galvan, A., Hare, T., Voss, H., Glover, G., & Casey, B. (2006). Risk taking and the adolescent brain: Who is at risk? *Developmental Science, 10*(2), F8–F14.

Herrman, J. (2005). The teen brain as a work in progress: Implications for pediatric nurses. *Pediatric Nursing, 31,* 144–148.

Johnson, S. B., Sudhinaraset, M., & Blum, R. W. (2010). Neuromaturation and adolescent risk taking: Why development is not determinism. *Journal of Adolescent Research, 25*(1), 4–23.

Males, M. (2009). Does the adolescent brain make risk taking inevitable? *Journal of Adolescent Research, 24*(1), 3–20.

McNeely, C., & Blanchard, J. (2009). *The teen years explained: A guide to healthy adolescent development.* Baltimore, MD: Johns Hopkins Bloomburg School of Public Health.

Selekman, J. (2008). Gambling: Normal adolescent activity or pathologic addiction? *Pediatric Nursing, 34*(4), 325–328.

Spear, L. P. (2000). Neurobehavioral changes in adolescence. *Current Directions in Psychological Science, 9*(4), 111–114.

Steinberg, L. (2004). Risk taking in adolescence: What changes and why? *Annals of the New York Academy of Science, 1021,* 51–58.

Steinberg, L. (2007). Risk taking in adolescence: New perspectives from brain and behavioral science. *Current Directions in Psychological Science, 16*(2), 55–59.

Steinberg, L., O'Brien, L., Cauffman, E., Graham, S., Woolard, J., & Banich, M. (2009). Age differences in future orientation and delay discounting. *Child Development, 80*(1), 28–44.

Van der Graff, J., Branje, S., DeWeid, M., Hawk, S., VanLier, P. V., & Meeus, W. (2013). Perspective taking and empathic concern in adolescence: Gender differences in developmental changes. *Developmental Psychology*. Advanced online publication. doi:10.1037/a0034325

Weinberger, D. R., Elevag, B., & Giedd, J. N. (2005). *The teen brain: A work in progress*. Washington, DC: The National Campaign to Prevent Teen and Unplanned Pregnancy.

Yurgelun-Todd, D. (2003). *Frontline interview: Inside the teen brain*. Retrieved from http://www.pbs.org

SUGGESTED WEBSITES

Kids Health.Org
www.kidshealth.org/teen

Advocates for Youth
www.advocatesforyouth.org

The National Campaign to Prevent Teen and Unplanned Pregnancy
www.nationalcampaign.org

Johns Hopkins School of Public Health
www.jhsph.edu

The Search Institute
www.search-institute.org

The Partnership at Drugfree.org
www.teenbrain.drugfree.org

National Institute of Mental Health
www.nimh.nih.org

Public Broadcast System—*Frontline*
www.pbs.org/wgbh/pages/frontline/shows

3

Teens and Their Health

Working with teens to enhance their health requires that we examine today's teens and how we can best assist them on their road to adulthood. The happiness and health of children and teens are direct predictors of the health of a society. In fact, teens with a positive outlook on life and a feeling of well-being are more likely to be healthy as adults and to subscribe to fewer risk behaviors than those who are more pessimistic about their future.

In this chapter, you will learn to:

1. Discuss selected demographics that describe today's teens
2. Identify key health issues and trends impacting teens' health today
3. Discuss how teens' perceptions of health, peers, and family influences may impact their health status and receipt of health care
4. Identify key focused interventions based upon learned concepts

TODAY'S TEENS

There are estimated to be over 1 billion teens in the world—the largest number in world history—with 63 million residing in the United States. Today about 32% of the United States' population are less than 20 years of age while, in 2080, less than 20% will be in this cohort. Essentially, as the life expectancy increases, fewer teens will make up society. Despite their minority in our population, they represent the important next productive generation.

FAST FACTS in a NUTSHELL

Facts about today's teens in the United States:

- 51% of teens are girls; 49% are boys
- 60% of the adolescent population is non-Hispanic White, 17% non-Hispanic Black, 18% Hispanic, 4% Asian/Pacific Islander, and 1% American Indian
- 20% of teens are uninsured
- 22% of teens live in poverty; 10% live in "deep" poverty

Teens at greatest health risk in the coming years will be those living in poverty, having social disadvantage, and from ethnic minority backgrounds. The number of youth living in these circumstances will continue to grow and these teens may be the most vulnerable to health risks. Individuals of Hispanic origin represent the fastest growing subset in America. As political, economic, and social resources are analyzed, we will need to advocate for teens.

TEEN HEALTH

On the one hand, teens are relatively healthy and often have little need for health intervention.

- A strong heart, healthy muscles, and a body suffering little wear-and-tear often function quite well without intervention.
- A healthy immune system assists in avoiding infectious processes.
- This is the age group that has little need for management of chronic illness; instead, care is focused on health surveillance and health promotion as teens set down health behaviors that last a lifetime.
- Lifestyle habits related to nutrition, sleep, exercise, stress management, and balance are created during the teen years.
- Teens may take their good health for granted. Since their health status has generally been good, they may not consider threats to their health as seriously as adults.
- Addressing teen health is critical before inappropriate health habits become deeply ingrained and difficult to change, as with smoking or nutritional patterns. Based on this fact alone, some consider that public health efforts should focus on adolescents.
- Allergies have emerged on the scene as significant pediatric and adolescent conditions requiring ongoing care and surveillance.
- Those teens with chronic illness require ongoing care. Young people with serious chronic illness are experiencing greater survival rates and health care providers are learning how to care for adults with conditions that were previously considered pediatric in nature.
- Researchers demonstrate that efforts directed toward prevention and early intervention during the teen years with such issues as obesity, essential hypertension, cancer, and avoidance of risk behaviors are warranted.

On the other hand:

- Adolescence is a time when there is a reduction in supervision of daily health practices by parents.
- Teens lack understanding of the impact today's actions will impose on later health.

- Teens engage in riskier behaviors that often threaten health.
- Adolescents tend not to seek out health care unless directed by an adult.
- Teens may distrust or devalue health care based on such factors as lack of confidentiality, cost, transportation, lack of teen-friendly components, need for parental consent or for parents to be informed via insurance or payment mechanisms, and lack of developmentally appropriate resources.
- One study noted that about 60% of young teens reported having a primary care visit in the past year, with this percentage decreasing as teens in the study aged.

As discussed, risk behaviors also pose a threat to teen health. For example, use of alcohol, drugs, and tobacco, along with unsafe sexual and interpersonal behaviors, all place teens at risk for harm or health issues. Several theories attempt to explain teens' attraction to risk behavior and desire for "thrills." How adolescents care for their bodies, engage in risk behaviors, and develop health habits will also have impact on future health. Table 3.1 depicts potential reasons teens may engage in high-risk behaviors.

TABLE 3.1 Why Teens Participate in High-Risk Behaviors

Adolescent brain development	Hormonal influences
Dopamine-induced sensation seeking	Personality and disposition differences
Genetic predisposition	Learning behaviors or disabilities
To gain control over their lives	To achieve adult status
Asynchronous pubertal maturation	In imitation of role model behaviors
To exert independence	To express opposition to authority
To be defiant	To deal with anxiety
To gain acceptance or recognition from others	To confirm individual identity

TABLE 3.2 Influences on Teen Health Behaviors

Gender	Attitudes	Religiosity
Family structure	Social content	Resources
Ethnicity	Culture	Self-esteem
Knowledge	Peer pressure	Personal resilience
Parental monitoring	Family connectedness	Role models
Parenting style	Family communication style	Socioeconomic status
Media	Music	Siblings

TEEN PERCEPTIONS OF HEALTH

The perceptions of teens about health and its priority may impact teen health behaviors. Teens associate health with the ability to participate in sports and activities, popularity, and physical attractiveness. Teens also noted that appropriate levels of sleep and optimal nutrition were associated with health. Less-identified elements included lifestyle risk behaviors, sexual risk behaviors, and stress. In addition, teens viewed threats to health to include: suicidal ideations, violence, medical conditions, problems with peers or partners, problems at home, emotional issues, substance use, and injuries.

A variety of factors influence teen health behaviors. Some of these factors are found in Table 3.2.

THE POWER OF PEERS

- Peers are important influences on behavior and learning.
- The reliance on peers and peers' importance during the teens years may have evolutionary roots whereby depending upon others and mutual support enhanced the chances of survival.
- Although peer pressure is not unique to teens and persists throughout life, it is thought to be most

intense during the teen years. Peer pressure peaks between 14 and 18 years of age, and this influence may be more significant than any other influence confronting teens.

- Resources reinforce that peer influences, both positive and negative, have the most powerful impact on teens' engagement in adolescent health and risk behaviors.
- Teens tend to engage in risky behaviors in the presence of friends.
- Peers may have a positive impact on health by sharing information, encouraging positive behaviors, guiding friends through difficult circumstances, role modeling healthy practices, and providing feedback to promote health priorities. Peers have been noted to decrease stress levels and enhance self-esteem in comrades, increasing perceptions of health and well-being.
- Gender may impact this influence in that health behaviors in teen males may be perceived by peers as a positive; that is, healthy behaviors, such as working out, drinking water, and balancing life activities are thought to be positive and make young men more popular. Interestingly, healthy behaviors among young women are not always deemed as positive, wherein adherence to healthy practices, such as sports and good eating habits, may be deemed as obedience practices and reflect a lack of independence from adults and others.

FAMILY INFLUENCES ON HEALTH

- The family also shapes adolescent views on health through the sharing of norms, attitudes, and behaviors.
- Families influence teen health behaviors and practices laid down early in life.
- Family connectedness, family structure, communication patterns, reinforcement of healthy habits, and role modeling influence teen health behaviors.

- Experts declare that, especially for teens considered at risk, "one concerned adult" can be a powerful force in reinforcing health behaviors.

HEALTH TRENDS AND PRIORITIES

As with other age groups, teens are largely healthier than ever before. Longer life expectancies may be impacted by healthier childhoods and adolescent periods. In contrast, there are some areas of teen health that have deteriorated or, at least, have not improved. Although the mortality rate has fallen in the past 3 decades for most age groups, it has actually remained steady or only slowly declined among 15- to 24-year-olds. The three most prominent causes of death among teens are unintentional accidents and motor vehicle accidents, homicide, and suicide. In fact, three quarters of the deaths among teens are from these three causes. Significant cultural and ethnic differences characterize these statistics, warranting specific interventions directed toward those groups at greatest risk. The primary teen risk behaviors are noted in Table 3.3.

Assessment of adolescent health status revealed that the teen mortality rate is declining, teens perceive higher levels of health and report fewer health limitations, and more teens report living in a smoke-free environment than previous cohorts of teens. In contrast, fewer teens report a healthy weight than those in previous years. Obesity levels across the life span are much higher than in the past and are currently on the rise in America. Globally, motor vehicle accidents,

TABLE 3.3 Teen Risk Behaviors

Alcohol and drug abuse	Intentional and unintentional injuries
Tobacco use	Unsafe sexual behaviors
Unhealthy dietary or eating patterns	Physical inactivity

suicides, homicides, and infectious diseases, including AIDS, dominate the mortality statistics. Teens are especially vulnerable to mental health issues.

- Trauma and stressful events may impact mental health for a lifetime.
- There are greater numbers of teens with mental health issues than ever before and yet data reveal that only about half are diagnosed and managed.
- Many psychopathologies emerge during the teen years, including depression, schizophrenia, anxiety, and personality disorder.
- Supports, or the lack thereof, provided during teen years to deal with crisis, stress, and trauma may have persistent impacts throughout the life of the individual.
- One study revealed that one third of teens attempting to receive mental health care withdrew their request in fear that their parents would be notified.
- Mental health issues render a significant toll on the lives of teens and their families.

In previous years, communicable illnesses posed the greatest threats to mankind. Interestingly, a recent perusal of the major health threats impacting teens highlights that priorities in teen health tend to be psychosocial in origin, wherein lifestyle choices, risk, and decision-making dominate teen health concerns. This sets the teen years apart from other ages in which illness, physical vulnerability, communicability, and chronicity dominate health issues. These major health issues, as articulated in the Critical National Health Objectives, are found in Table 3.4.

In order to address the unique needs of teens, we must focus on risk assessment, education of both parents and teens, anticipatory guidance, prevention, and support for positive health behaviors while moving away from the traditional health care model of screening, diagnosis, and treatment of disease.

TABLE 3.4 Trends in Critical National Health Objectives for Adolescents and Young Adults

Objective	Change From Baseline	Subgroups of Concern
Overall mortality: Reduce deaths	No change (except Black males—worsened)	Males, Blacks
Reduce deaths by motor vehicle crashes	No change	Males, Whites
Reduce deaths by alcohol-related motor vehicle crashes	Improved	Males, Hispanics
Increase use of seatbelts	Improved	Males, Blacks
Reduce number of teens who report riding with a driver drinking alcohol	Improved	Males, Hispanics
Reduce homicides	Improved	Males, Blacks
Reduce physical fighting	Improved	Males, Blacks
Reduce weapon carrying at school	Improved	Males, Hispanics
Reduce suicide rates	Improved	Male, Whites
Reduce suicide attempts requiring medical attention	No change	Females, Hispanics
Reduce binge drinking	Worsened	Males, Whites
Reduce use of illicit substances (marijuana)	Worsened	Males, Whites
Reduce number of children with disabilities who report they are sad, unhappy, or depressed	Improved	Females, Blacks
Increase number of children with mental health issues who receive treatment	No change	Females, Hispanics
Reduce pregnancies in teen females	Improved	Blacks
Reduce new HIV diagnoses	No change	Not available
Increase number of teens who never had intercourse	No change	Males, Blacks
Increase number of teens who are not currently sexually active	Worsened	Females, Blacks
Increase number of sexually active teens who use condoms	No change	Females, Hispanics

(continued)

TABLE 3.4 Trends in Critical National Health Objectives for Adolescents and Young Adults (*continued*)

Objective	Change From Baseline	Subgroups of Concern
Reduce incidence of *Chlamydia* infections	Worsened	Males, Blacks
Increase females attending family planning clinics	Worsened	Blacks
Increase females attending sexually transmitted infections (STI) clinics	Worsened	Blacks
Increase males attending STI clinics	Worsened	Blacks
Reduce tobacco use	Improved	Male, Whites
Reduce obesity and overweight	Worsened	Males, Hispanics
Increase teens who engage in physical activity	No change	Females, Blacks

Adapted from Jiang et al. (2011)

FOCUSED INTERVENTIONS

- Be vigilant of the primary health care needs of teens as they progress through the adolescent years.
- Rely on the power of peers to guide interventions, including peer mentors, role models, and leaders.
- Use each interface with teens as an opportunity for a brief intervention. These may include assessment (Why? What? How? How long? When?) and provision of information about safe alternatives.
- Motivational interviewing is a higher-level educational process, often requiring special training, wherein individuals are asked to reflect on habits, reasons for habits, consequences of habits, alternatives to habits, consequences of alternatives, and means to change behavior. The four key elements of motivational interviewing include: expressing empathy, developing discrepancy, rolling with resistance, and supporting self-efficacy.

- Another framework applies the principles of risk reduction to teens such that they: become aware of the risk and threats to their health, come to realize their personal vulnerability, modify their beliefs, change their behavior, and are able to access and afford health-protective alternatives that foster positive behavior change.
- Harm-reduction principles stipulate that any decrease in risk behavior results in a positive, if not total, decrease in risk. For example, smoking fewer cigarettes, using condoms on even days during sexual activity, drinking to excess only when at home, or smoking marijuana only after school characterize harm reduction principles. Although controversial, many ascribe to harm reduction as an alternative to total behavior change, which can easily lapse to previous risk behaviors.

SUGGESTED READING

Berryman, P. S. (2012). *Reducing teen and unplanned pregnancy to strengthen the future workforce.* Washington, DC: National Business Group on Health.

Burstein, G. R., Lowry, R., Klein, J. D., & Santelli, J. S. (2003). Missed opportunities for sexually transmitted diseases, HIV, and pregnancy prevention services during adolescent health supervision visits. *Pediatrics, 111*, 996–1001.

ChildTrends. (2013). *What do we know about the high school class of 2013?* Retrieved from http://www.childtrends.org

Christopherson, T. M., & Jordan-Marsh, M. (2004). Culture and risk-taking in adolescents' behavior. *MCN: The American Journal of Maternal/Child Nursing, 29*, 100–105.

Cohall, A. T., Cohall, R., Dye, B., Din, S., Vaughan, R. D., & Coots, S. (2007). Overheard in the halls: What adolescents are saying and what teachers are saying about health issues. *Journal of School Health, 77*, 344–350.

DiClemente, R. J., Santelli, J. S., & Crosby, R. A. (Eds.). (2009). *Adolescent health: Understanding and prevention risk behaviors.* San Francisco, CA: Jossey-Bass.

Eaton, D. K., Kann, L., Kinchen, S., Shanklin, S., Flint, K. H., Hawkins, J., . . . Wechsler, H. (2012). Youth risk behavior surveillance—United States, 2011. *MMWR, 61*(4), 1–162.

Henderson, A., & Champlin, S. (1998). *Promoting teen health.* Thousand Oaks, CA: Sage.

Hoyt, L. T., Chase-Lansdale, P., McDade, T. W., & Adams, E. K. (2012). Positive youth, healthy adults: Does positive well-being in adolescence predict better perceived health and fewer risky behaviors in young adulthood? *Journal of Adolescent Health, 50,* 66–73.

Jiang, N., Kolbe, L. J., Seo, D. C., Kay, N. S., & Brindis, C. D. (2011). Health of adolescents and young adults: Trends in achieving the 21 critical National Health Objectives by 2010. *Journal of Adolescent Health, 49,* 124–132.

Ma, J., Wang, Y., & Stafford, R. S. (2005). US adolescents receive suboptimal preventive counseling during ambulatory care. *Journal of Adolescent Health, 36,* 441.

Marcell, A. V., & Halpern-Felsher, B. L. (2007). Adolescent beliefs about preferred resources for help vary depending on the health issue. *Journal of Adolescent Health, 41,* 61–68.

Miller, W. R., & Rollnick, S. (2002). *Motivational interviewing: Preparing people for change.* New York, NY: Guilford Press.

Mulye, T. P., Park, M. J., Nelson, C. D., Adams, S. H., Irwin, C. E., & Brindis, C. D. (2009). Trends in adolescent and young adult health in the US. *Journal of Adolescent Health, 45,* 8–24.

National Institute for Health Care Management Research and Education Foundation (NIHCM). (2011). *Protecting confidential health services for adolescents & young adults: Strategies and considerations for health plans.* Washington, DC: Author.

Ott, M. A., Rosenberg, J. G., McBride, K. R., & Woodcox, S. G. (2011). How do adolescents view health? Implications for state health policy. *Journal of Adolescent Health, 48,* 398–403.

Roy, K., Hadden, A. G., Ikeda, R. M., Curry, C. W., Truman, B. I., & Thacker, S. B. (2009). Monitoring progress toward CDC's health protection goals: Health outcome measures by life stage. *Public Health Reports, 124,* 304–316.

Steinberg, L. (2004). Risk taking in adolescence: What changes and why? *Annals of the New York Academy of Science, 1021,* 51–58.

Steinberg, L. (2008). *Adolescence.* New York, NY: McGraw-Hill.

SUGGESTED WEBSITES

Kids Health.Org
www.kidshealth.org/teen
Healthy Teen Network
www.healthyteennetwork.org
Children's Hospital of Boston
www.childrenshospital.org
Go Ask Alice
www.goaskalice.columbia.edu
Johns Hopkins School of
Public Health
www.jhsph.edu
Girl Scouts
www.girlscouts.org
AddHealth
www.cpc.unc.edu/projects/
addhealth
Child Trends
www.childtrends.org

The Urban Institute
www.urban.org
Kaiser Foundation
www.kff.org
Centers for Disease Control
and Prevention
www.cdc.gov/healthyyouth
National Center for Health
Statistics
www.cdc.gov/nchs
American Medical Association
www.ama-assn.org
Society for Adolescent
Medicine and Health
www.adolescenthealth.org
Healthy People
www.healthypeople.gov

4

Working With Teens

Working with teens warrants special skills in developing partnerships, and communicating with and understanding teens. Despite the fact that teens approach adults' physical size, their health decision-making may not be mature enough to manage their own health surveillance and health practices.

Teens' sensation-seeking, difficulty in delaying impulses, susceptibility to peer pressure, and lack of cognitive controls not only predispose them to high-risk behaviors but also to poor daily choices as far as healthy eating, sleep habits, participation in exercise, hobbies, coping with stress, and other interests that allow for a balanced life. The need for consequences of actions and behaviors to be relevant, immediately applicable, and visible or tangible will impact how teens interpret health teaching and embrace health behaviors.

In this chapter, you will learn to:

1. Discuss how adults and teens may partner to optimize teen health
2. List several health care providers working with teens
3. Identify principles to promote effective communication with teens
4. Identify key focused interventions based upon learned concepts

TEENS AS PARTNERS IN HEALTH DECISION-MAKING

Recent studies tell us that teens want to be considered partners in their health care, along with caring, knowledgeable, and consistent adults. Decision-making skills developed during the teen years may impact future health, health-seeking behaviors, and health priorities. Teens' difficulties in processing abstract concepts, such as communicability of infections, malignancy, long-term consequences, and the relationship of behaviors to health, may all contribute to teens' adherence to recommended health practices. The teen decision-making process may be considered impulsive or rational, as differentiated in Table 4.1.

If teen decision-making is rational, then...

- Providing information to teens about healthy patterns would logically lead to healthier behaviors.
- Much of our prevention agenda directed toward teens, especially related to health and risk behaviors, would be based on the provision of information and supplies and making assumptions on how teens will respond.
- But, just knowing about healthy lifestyles and fostering health does not always translate to behavior change or adopting habits known to be healthy.

TABLE 4.1 Are Teens Impulsive or Rational?

Impulsive	Rational
Unconscious	Conscious
Spontaneous	Deliberate consideration of consequences
Peer and media influenced	Independent
Impacted by substance use	Weighing of pros and cons
Immature	Mature
Concrete	Abstract
Reactive	Proactive
"If it feels good, do it"	Responsible

- Decision-making occurs in response to personal desires for pleasure, peer pressure, the desire to seek new and different sensations, or to express individuality.
- The direction of our prevention efforts warrants high levels of parental control and focusing efforts on parents as role models, supervisors, and monitors of health behavior, and creating alternative mechanisms in the absence of parents.

More likely, teen decision-making is neither completely impulsive nor deliberate, but a developmental process where, as teens mature, they become more able to participate in higher levels of cognitive function, become more independent in their own health surveillance, and temper their personal need for rewards and sensational experiences. New research about the characteristics of adolescent reasoning suggests that not all teens reach abstract reasoning during the teen years and that some adults never reach abstract reasoning. This lack of ability to comprehend abstract concepts has clear implications for health decision-making as teens navigate complex concepts of the human body and behavior.

The adult supervision required earlier in adolescence may make way for more progressive abilities to make personal choices about behaviors and lifestyle. Each adolescent must be assessed for his or her personal ability to assume responsibilities for health decision-making and must be provided the age-appropriate support for progressively more complex tasks. As they develop higher level skills, teens may be given the opportunity to make more complex choices and to consider increasingly intricate decisions about their health and health care.

Inherent to this model is the need for parental, guardian, or other adult presence, especially early in a teen's years, to offer support, information, and access to services, in addition to serving as a role model in healthy living. Parents and other family members need the information, confidence, and time to provide such support to teens. In homes where parents are unable to provide such support, whether due to personal issues, work and other obligations, home stresses, or other factors, outside sources can often provide the guidance teens need to be successful.

HEALTH CARE PROVIDERS

A variety of health care providers (HCPs) work with teens to foster positive health and health behaviors; some examples are given in Table 4.2.

Some teens continue with pediatricians and pediatric office staff until they reach 18 years of age. Others begin with or transition to adult or general practice offices along with other family members. Young women wanting reproductive health care may seek out gynecologists for assessments and provision of birth control. Teens of lower income may use publicly or privately subsidized clinics to obtain health care. Another area often forgotten is the importance of dental care and examinations. Public dental services for indigent populations including teens are gaining prevalence as we realize the impact of oral care on total body health.

A recent study of teen preferences for sources of health care, HCPs, and health information revealed that their opinions may be influenced by the type of health care needed and how teens interpret the resource's ability to meet that need. Teens identified physicians and medical clinics as

TABLE 4.2 Health Care Providers Working With Teens

Nurses	Physicians
Nurse practitioners	Physician assistants
School nurses	Respiratory/physical/occupational therapists
Social workers	Clergy
Health/physical education/ other teachers	Coaches/trainers
Music/art/other therapists	Speech pathologists
Counselors	Dentists
Psychologists	Dieticians/nutritionists

A new recommendation for young women is the omission of the need for teens to have a pelvic exam in order to receive oral or long-acting reversible contraceptives such as Depo-Provera, the pill, or the patch. It is recommended that young women receive a pelvic exam for screening at or before 21 years of age or within 3 years of becoming sexually active. The pelvic exam is often a deterrent for young women seeking birth control and this change in practice has been heralded as an important teen-friendly revision.

appropriate sources for health care related to injuries or illness. They sought out peers, family members, or partners for lifestyle issues, such as reproductive care and cigarette smoking. Mental health issues created the biggest quandary for teens because although they knew they should seek professional help, teens questioned the confidentiality and quality of the sources of mental health care in their world. The study sample resorted to peer consultation even though they knew professional help was indicated. Identifying the barriers to health care, as delineated in Table 4.3, may assist in efforts to alleviate those obstacles for teens.

Teens may also see HCPs in school-based health centers (SBHCs). These health care sites often include nurse practitioners, physician's assistants, social workers, counselors, dieticians, and others to provide holistic care in a school setting.

TABLE 4.3 Barriers to Teens' Access to Health Care

Transportation and location	Cost
Need for parental consent	Insurance issues and parental notification
Issues with privacy of medical records	Concern over confidentiality
Lack of teen-friendly services	Difficulties with hours and appointments

FAST FACTS in a NUTSHELL

- There are 1,930 SBHCs in 46 of the 50 states and six in the District of Columbia.
- 81% of SBHCs polled used teen feedback to guide their practices and 50% had youth advisory boards.
- Researchers demonstrate that SBHCs save significant monies in preventive health, reduce emergency room visits and hospitalizations, reduce teen pregnancy, decrease absenteeism and dropout, and have other positive outcomes.

- SBHCs are easily accessible, teen friendly, convenient, and generally free of cost. They provide important services to teens in such areas as assessment, management, education, and follow-up.
- SBHC services vary significantly among sites and may include health screening and referral, counseling and mental health services, nutrition services, health and sports physicals, and reproductive health services.
- Perhaps the greatest impacts of SBHCs in their public health goals of health promotion and disease prevention are the ability to screen, manage, educate, and follow up with services and assist teens in engaging in positive health behaviors and behavior change.
- Some SBHCs have expanded to provide services to other siblings, parents, extended family members, and community members, filling a critical need for the provision of primary health care.
- SBHCs work in collaboration with school nurses and individuals' medical homes, if they exist, to meet the needs of teen clients.
- SBHCs engage parents in SBHC advisory boards, in decisions about their children's health, and in educational efforts.

Communicating with teens has probably held challenges for generations. Technology added another level of reach and complexity as phones, computers, and other devices have broadened the scope of communication and allowed for social media to expand the breadth of human interaction.

Common Principles for Communicating With Teens

- As always, honesty is always the best policy. Teens may be astute to untruths or the communicator's discomfort with certain topics, increasing the potential for distrust and future wariness.
- Speak with teens on their terms. Teens may find times "good" for them to ventilate that don't always meet your schedule. It is important to remain flexible and approach topics on the teen's time frame to encourage free sharing of ideas.
- Clarify meanings and make sure you validate communication along the way. Don't get hung up on new words or new meanings for words. On the other hand, make sure you understand the teen's intent. I will never forget the day my son said a new dress I was wearing was "sick." As a nurse for many years, I needed to clarify that being "sick" was actually a good thing!
- Use "I" statements when talking with teens to avoid putting teens on the defensive. Saying "you" tends to make people feel vulnerable and attacked and will inhibit communication. Use a calm, noncondescending voice to establish assertiveness without aggressive tendencies.
- Use common principles of communication to portray sincerity, authenticity, and caring. Verbal and nonverbal cues, such as eye contact and gestures, go a long way. Make sure you read the signals of those with whom you are communicating and consider the impact of such cues on the message.

- Privacy is critical during the teen years, especially about sensitive subjects. Determining what is sensitive is also critical. Ensure that you are alone, or as alone as possible, when discussing private matters. This is especially important if peers may witness situations that may be embarrassing or infringe on privacy.
- Confidentiality is also a priority for teens. Make sure you are explicit about conditional confidentiality, wherein you will need to divulge information that indicates that the teen could harm himself or herself or others. Ensure that teens understand that this policy is designed for their safety and that of others.
- In today's environment, privacy may not always be available. "Two-deep" confrontations, designed to avoid exploitation or potentially difficult situations, may change the dynamics of the interaction. Explaining policies and the need for these practices will enable teens to adapt to current changes.
- Communicate consequences to teens in honest, unbiased, and positive terms.
- Discuss one topic at a time to avoid confusion and ensure comprehension.
- Set ground rules for communication based on mutual respect. Do not sacrifice your personal principles but be open about each others' needs and preferences.
- Be astute to potential reasons behind teens' behaviors or communication patterns. Negativity, lack of kindness, or insensitivity may be cover-ups for discomfort or poor self-esteem.
- Confronting difficult topics can be a challenge for teens. When conducting an assessment or collecting data, always start with the least sensitive concepts first and proceed to the more sensitive topics. This allows you to build trust.
- If you don't know an answer to a question, don't punt! Look it up, research it together, or discuss potential alternatives.
- Use open-ended questions with teens. Teens find it easy to say "yes" or "no" without much depth. Probing questions may be needed to elicit comprehensive information.

- Honesty and respect are critical in establishing partnerships with teens about health care.
- Consider your local area and the health care services available. Determine if there are gaps in health resources or barriers to care for teens. Advocate for teen-focused care that addresses these gaps and barriers.
- Allow teens graduated opportunities for decision-making and encourage independence as teens develop.
- Clarify the roles of HCPs with teens and help them to navigate the complex health care system as needed.
- Remember their developmental levels when communicating and working with teens about their health and health care.

SUGGESTED READING

Clayton, S., Chin, R., Blackburn, S., & Echeverria, C. (2010). Different setting, different care: Integrating prevention and clinical care in school-based health centers. *American Journal of Public Health, 100*, 1592–1596.

Feinstein, S. (2007). *Teaching the at-risk teenage brain*. Lanham, MD: Rowman & Littlefield.

Herrman, J. W. (2007). Repeat pregnancy in adolescence: Intentions and decision making. *MCN: The American Journal of Maternal/Child Nursing, 32*(2), 89–94.

School-Based Health Alliance. (2014). *2010–2011 census report*. Washington, DC: Author.

Spear, L. P. (2000). Neurobehavioral changes in adolescence. *Current Directions in Psychological Science, 9*(4), 111–114.

Steinberg, L. (2004). Risk taking in adolescence: What changes and why? *Annals of the New York Academy of Science, 1021*, 51–58.

Steinberg, L. (2007). Risk taking in adolescence: New perspectives from brain and behavioral science. *Current Directions in Psychological Science, 16*(2), 55–59.

Steinberg, L., & Manahan, K. C. (2007). Age differences in resistance to peer influence. *Developmental Psychology, 43*(6), 1531–1543.

Sutherland, P. (1999). The application of Piagetian and neo-Piagetian ideas to further and higher education. *International Journal of Lifelong Education, 18,* 286–295.

SUGGESTED WEBSITES

Kids Health.Org
www.kidshealth.org/teen
Advocates for Youth
www.advocatesforyouth.org
SEICUS
www.seicus.org
The Urban Institute
www.urban.org
The Bureau For At-Risk Youth
www.at-risk.com
Children's Hospital of Boston
www.childrenshospital.org

American Medical Association
www.ama-assn.org
Society for Adolescent
Medicine and Health
www.adolescenthealth.org
Healthy People
www.healthypeople.gov
Johns Hopkins School of
Public Health
www.jhsph.edu
School-Based Health Alliance
www.sbh4all.org

Adolescent Health Domains

5

Physical Health and Risks

Often it is the physical characteristics of children and adolescents that we notice first. Their growth, acquisition of adult traits, and rapid changes are very visible and are measures by which we assess maturation, nutritional status, exposure to stimulation, and care. Physical health is impacted by health patterns and risk behaviors.

In this chapter, you will learn to:

1. Explore selected aspects of the assessment of physical development
2. Analyze key issues, including nutrition, obesity, eating disorders, physical fitness, sleep, and sports, as they impact physical health
3. Discuss risk behaviors, such as those associated with body decoration and unintentional injuries, as they impact teen health
4. Identify key focused interventions based upon learned concepts

PHYSICAL DEVELOPMENT

- Developmental assessment of a teen occurs more from a report and history basis, rather than by witnessing the mastery of selected large and gross motor milestones as done in childhood.
- Teens' abilities in sports, their coordination, reports of progress in school, observation during time spent with the teen, and soliciting the concerns of teens and families about physical development all contribute to this assessment.
- Screenings, such as vision, hearing, scoliosis, dental, environmental/disease exposure, and immunization records, all provide information about physical development and health.
- Measurement of height and weight and calculations of body mass index (BMI) give health care providers (HCPs) an idea about the teen's physical size, determine how these measurements rank with norms and percentiles, and yield impressions about growth and body weight.

FAST FACTS in a NUTSHELL

Sometime during adolescence most teens experience an adolescent growth spurt such that the teen reaches a peak growth velocity of 3 to 4 inches per year and gains one-half of his or her body weight. This occurs 2 years earlier in girls than it does in boys.

The Tanner stages provide an assessment of the assumption of secondary sex characteristics and a means to compare chronological age, sexual development, and societal norms. The Tanner scale is used to assess both boys and girls during puberty (Table 5.1).

Significant attention has been devoted to the achievement of puberty, how this timing compares with the teen's chronological age, and the issues arising from early and late maturation. Table 5.2 compares selected issues associated with early and late maturing.

TABLE 5.1 Tanner Stages of Sexual Development

Tanner Stage	Breast Development	Penile Development	Pubic Hair Development
1	No breast development	Slight increase in penis size but no change from childhood appearance	No pubic hair
2	Breast buds	Scrotum enlarges, changes in color and texture of scrotal skin	Small amount of long, straight pubic hair
3	More distinct breast tissue	Increase in penis length	Small amount of darker, curlier pubic hair
4	Breast enlargement, secondary enlargement of areola	Increase in length and breadth of the penis with further maturation of the scrotum	Adult-type hair but only covers a small area of the pubis
5	Breast fully developed, areola recedes into contour of breast	Penis and scrotum adult in shape and characteristics	Adult-type hair, spreads to form an inverse triangle

TABLE 5.2 Early- and Late-Maturing Teens

Early-Maturing Teens	Late-Maturing Teens
Teens who achieve early puberty and appear older than their chronological age may experience different stressors, including increased demands, sustained interactions with older peers, and early sexual maturation	Teens attaining puberty later than the norm and, potentially, their peers may have concerns about their development and require assurance that their development will be similar to their peers but on their own timeline

(continued)

TABLE 5.2 Early- and Late-Maturing Teens (*continued*)

Early-Maturing Teens	Late-Maturing Teens
Early-maturing boys may be treated favorably with their newly acquired height and stature, whereas girls may feel gawky and self-conscious	Late-maturing individuals may lack in confidence or experience decreased self-esteem
More precocious teens are more prone to participate in high-risk behaviors, are frequently expected to act older than their chronological age, and may be victims of exploitation because their cognitive controls may not be developed or ready to deal with issues confronted during the teen years	Youths with smaller body size and muscle mass may use anabolic steroids to increase the size of body muscle. It is estimated that 3%–9% of teens use anabolic steroids, with use peaking in the middle school years. The associated health risks include stimulating aggression, physiologic changes in organ function, mood alterations, emotional lability, and potential decreased cognitive function

FAST FACTS in a NUTSHELL

- Many teens have dietary patterns that result in deficiencies in protein, fiber, and valuable calories and excesses in sodium, fats, and empty calories.
- Only 20% of teens report eating 5 or more fruits and vegetables per day, with about 6% of students reporting eating no vegetables and 5% no fruit.
- Almost half of teens, when asked if they were trying to lose weight, indicated they were currently on or just went off a restrictive diet, and 60% of teens reported they exercised to lose or keep from gaining weight in the 30 days prior to the survey.
- Of greater concern, 12% fasted for more than 24 hours and 6% took diet pills to lose or to keep from gaining weight.

NUTRITION

Nutrition is a concern of every generation. Economics, life-style, tradition, and family practices may dictate nutritional choices that are not based on current knowledge of optimal eating practices. The teen years are often a time to divert from learned nutritional practices, follow peers in their dietary choices, and sustain increased nutritional demands related to growth, activity, and development.

Concern about fast food, soda and empty-calorie beverages, readily available snack foods, and less availability of fresh fruits and vegetables informs current advocacy efforts. Increasing emphasis on the importance of frequent meals, especially breakfast, led to the provision of meals in schools. Campaigns to withdraw selected foods and beverages from schools, the availability of caloric charts in restaurants, and increased emphasis on increasing the numbers of fruits and vegetables in the daily diet were launched to foster better nutrition.

- Although there has been significant attention on the questionable eating habits of teens, some sources indicate that the teen years may be a time when individuals demonstrate high levels of nutrition. Some teens today drink adequate amounts of water, choose healthy alternatives at meals, and prefer snacks that are healthy and satisfying.
- Although some authorities feel that multivitamins are not needed in clients who have adequate intake of all nutrients, the increased physical growth and potential for nutritional deficits lead many experts to recommend daily multivitamins for teens. Some young women also need iron, which should be monitored by a physician or nurse practitioner.
- Obviously, much of teen nutrition is related to family practices, the availability of nutritious food, and support for nutrition.
- Habits such as eating a healthy breakfast, ensuring adequate intake of fresh or freshly cooked fruits and

vegetables, limiting processed foods, nutritious snacking, promoting family dinners and optimal nutritional patterns, and ensuring that the intake of calories is commensurate with caloric expenditure may begin and be reinforced during the teen years.

OVERWEIGHT AND OBESITY

Some of those issues leading to nutritional deficits or excesses may translate to obesity. Overweight and obesity are growing problems across the life span and are significant in some youth. These issues may set the stage for a lifetime of overweight issues.

FAST FACTS in a NUTSHELL

By definition, overweight individuals are in the 85% percentile and obesity is for those in the 95%. About 31% of teens nationwide are considered overweight or obese, which is close to four times the rate of 40 years ago. Selected ethnic groups are at increased risk for obesity, with Black females and Black and Hispanic males especially at risk. Eighty percent of obese adolescents will become obese adults.

Issues with overconsumption of calories, increased sugar and fat intake, compulsive eating, low fiber intake, large portions of food, inadequate physical activity to burn calories, calorie-dense foods that do not satiate the appetite, genetic factors, and biological differences in metabolism may all contribute to the development of obesity. Obesity and overweight may lead to health issues such as metabolic syndrome, type 2 diabetes, sleep apnea, joint and bone disorders, cardiovascular disease, and functional health problems. Negative social and psychoemotional issues include problems with peers, poor self-esteem, rejection, body image stressors, stigma

TABLE 5.3 Effective Weight-Control Strategies

- Journaling daily food intake
- Cognitive-behavioral interventions
- Education about portions
- Increasing water consumption
- Programs on exercise, walking, and increasing daily activities
- Limiting of fast foods
- Group support for weight loss with online and social media monitoring and encouragement
- School-related interventions and limitation of food and beverage choices
- Behavioral therapy and medications
- Family-focused interventions emphasizing optimal nutrition, role modeling of positive behaviors, enhancing communication, providing an environment in which positive choices can be made, engaging in fitness, and feeling positive about one's body
- Community supports to foster family interventions
- Controversy exists over the use of gastric banding or surgical procedures for teens except in extreme cases

and prejudice, social isolation, anxiety, depression, and poor social competence. Financial implications compound these negative impacts, including care of chronic conditions, complications, and potential health care costs.

Prevention strategies for obesity include those focused on good nutrition and health, increasing activity, and investigation of the emotional and nonnutritional origins of eating. Many schools monitor the BMI of their students. Sending BMI report cards to parents supports recognition of vulnerability for problems associated with overweight and obesity, and encourages parents to address the issue. Table 5.3 includes strategies deemed to be effective in weight control.

EATING DISORDERS

A preoccupation with body type and quality is prominent across the life span in today's society. Feelings of inadequacy and concern with body image occur in both genders and in teens and adults. Of special concern with teens today are eating disorders such as anorexia nervosa and bulimia. Though they have similarities, they are characterized by fundamental differences that require different assessment and management. For both disorders, the need for counseling, family therapy, and understanding is paramount (Table 5.4).

TABLE 5.4 Anorexia Nervosa and Bulimia

	Anorexia Nervosa	Bulimia
Definition	Perceptions of overweight and distorted body image lead to extensive measures to lose weight Fear of gaining weight	Binge eating in response to stress or upset followed by purging and expressions of guilt
Behaviors	Cessation of eating Purging of food eaten by vomiting and use of cathartics Denying the need to eat Achievement-oriented personalities Extensive effort at meal preparation but refusing to eat Excessive exercise	Binging on large amount of food (usually a single food) Purging of food eaten via self-induced vomiting, use of laxatives, diuretics, exercise, or combinations thereof Behaviors usually done in secret Callouses may be noted on fingers
Age of onset/ gender	5% of females, 1% males Any race, most often White Peaks at 12–13 years and 17–18 years Leads to amenorrhea	5% or more, mostly young women; middle-to-late adolescence or college years Mostly in Western or westernized cultures
Etiology	May be associated with a significant stressor Many causes Chemical changes in the brain and blood have been noted	Associated with stress and the quest for body perfection Social pressures for thinness Family chaos or stress

(continued)

TABLE 5.4 Anorexia Nervosa and Bulimia *(continued)*

	Anorexia Nervosa	Bulimia
Consequences	Severe weight loss May be life-threatening Fluid and electrolyte imbalance Cardiac dysrhythmias	Normal or slightly overweight Electrolyte imbalances Dental erosions Gastroesophageal reflux disease Myocardial damage Dehydration
Treatment	Clinical therapy Focus on slow weight gain (not food eaten) Allow for control Behavior modification Hospitalization if 25%–30% below optimal body weight	Physical stabilization Cognitive retraining Very difficult to treat
Psychological manifestations	Depression Isolation Suicidal ideations	Fear, guilt, anxiety Loss of coping behaviors

Though males and females of any race can develop anorexia nervosa, it is found primarily in teen girls. Treatment for anorexia allows for progressive increases in food intake while reorienting the client to the realities of his or her body size and need for food. The course of anorexia often includes remissions and exacerbations and requires ongoing therapy and surveillance.

═══════════════════════*FAST FACTS in a NUTSHELL*

The "female athlete triad" has been identified, wherein young women who excel in sport, have high expectations for themselves, feel ambivalent about their bodies, and have perfectionistic qualities engage in anorexia behaviors.

Clients with bulimia may find early eating episodes pleasurable, but then the individuals may fear loss of control and weight gain. Although treatment can be difficult, the individual usually has an accurate body image and needs to learn alternate ways to cope with stress and conflict. Bulimia may recur at times of extreme stress. Binge-eating disorder is diagnosed in teens when binging occurs three or more times per week and is not compensated by purging.

FITNESS/EXERCISE

Adolescence is a time of growing physical coordination, eye–hand coordination, competitiveness, same-sex activities, and the need to "blow off steam." In addition to attaining and maintaining healthy weight and muscle mass, participation in sports and fitness is thought to enhance learning, the ability to manage stress, emotional control, and memory. Many teens get enough exercise during their participation in school sports, daily physical education classes, or with informal physical activities.

FAST FACTS in a NUTSHELL

- About 35% of teens reported getting the recommended physical activity (60 or more minutes/day, 5 times/week); this decreases to 22% for individuals 18 to 24 years of age.
- Previous recommendations of 30 minutes of exercise three times per week showed greater success, with 65% of teens meeting that benchmark.
- As society has become more sedentary and lost much of the need to walk to get places, fitness emerged as a concern across the life span.
- Thirty percent of teens reported playing video or computer games 3 or more hours a day, and the average "screen time" for teens is estimated at 6 hours per day.

TABLE 5.5 Suggestions for Acceptable Physical Activities

- Supporting teen recess such that teens get a break during the school day
- Bullying prevention activities that encourage full participation in sports and fitness activities
- Fostering daily physical education in schools throughout the entire school experience
- Promoting family activities that involve movement and exercise
- Normalization of walking in day-to-day activities

School districts that do not support daily physical education or do not have late buses to allow for sports, perhaps due to budget constraints, require encouragement to reconsider practices. Individuals who are low income, not involved in sports, rural, or from homes with less support tend to be especially impacted by these restrictions and may inordinately suffer from poor levels of fitness. Some girls feel that exercise or sports involvement may be unfeminine or unacceptable, warranting exploration of physical activities that work for everyone (Table 5.5).

SPORTS AND SPORTS INJURIES

About 8 million adolescents participate in sports annually. As noted, the teen years are a time when sports provide diversional activity, physical activity, stress management, peer contact, healthy competition, and teamwork. Some schools are unable to provide sports activities for all teens and advocates are encouraging schools and community groups to expand and diversify their sports to embrace all teens.

The most common, nonfatal sources of injuries in teens are sports injuries. The most common injuries occur in football, basketball, roller skating, and baseball. Several significant sports injuries have come into public attention in the past decade including concussions, soft tissue injuries, and orthopedic fractures, sprains, and strains. Person-to-person or object contact in sports has highlighted new concern related to concussions, the leading injury causing hospitalization, in such sports as hockey, horseback riding, skiing, soccer, and skateboarding. Injuries occurring as results of falls, impact with another player, overexertion, or being hit with an object have instigated legislation in many states related to updating and maintenance of sports equipment, coach education, prevention strategies (such as taping ankles), protocols for treatment after injuries, and time out of sports participation due to an injury. Treatment may include comfort measures, pain management, physical therapy, immobilization, or surgery. Although outside the scope of this text, education about prevention, safe sports equipment, monitoring of sportsman-like conduct, and enforcement of safety practices will prevent some sports injuries.

SLEEP

Teen brain development impacts other areas related to health and wellness, including teens' sleep behaviors. The average teen gets between 5 and 6 hours of sleep, despite the anticipated sleep needs of 9 hours or more per night (Table 5.6).

Most teens report that they suffer from insufficient sleep and rest. Teens' inabilities to fall sleep at an appropriate time,

---

TABLE 5.6 Factors Impacting Teen Sleep

- The pineal gland, found beneath the midbrain, is responsible for releasing melatonin, the neurotransmitter responsible for sleep. Melatonin signals to the brain how to "shut down" for sleep. Because of the lack of maturity in pineal function, teens need more time to fall asleep
- "Screen time" with computers, televisions, and other electronic devices delay melatonin secretion
- Late school activities, large volumes of homework, and work schedules impede sleep
- Lack of structured bedtimes, bedtime routines, and sleep hygiene (personal habits prior to sleep time that signal to the body that it is time to go to sleep) all contribute to sleep deprivation

early school times, and other demands may impair learning, cause vacillating moods, and potentially impact behavior. Sleep disorders such as sleepwalking, night terrors, insomnia, mental health issues related to sleep disturbances, and narcolepsy, though rare in adolescence, do occur in youth and often require intervention. Daytime sleepiness, reduced academic performance, and substance use may all figure into this generation of teens who are chronically fatigued. HCP interventions include screening, counseling, and teaching about sleep hygiene practices.

BODY DECORATION

Teens' tattoos and body piercings, similar to others across the life span, are manifestations of individuality and personal expression, peer influence, or having meaning in their ability to express an idea or membership in a group. Key to addressing body decoration is to leave bias or judgment out of the HCP intervention with teens. Instead, HCPs should consider the implications for such body decorations and to focus on the health and safety concerns associated with such practices (Table 5.7).

TABLE 5.7 Health Implications of Tattoos and Piercings

Tattoos	Piercings
Counseling prior to application—visibility, cost, location, and permanence	Counseling prior to application—visibility, cost, location, and permanence
Ensure that tattoos are personally desired, not based on influence or pressure from others	Ensure that piercings are personally desired, not based on influence or pressure from others
The reputability of the agency and its cleanliness/techniques should be considered	The reputability of the agency and its cleanliness/techniques should be considered. Home piercing is quite common; infection control procedures should be followed

(continued)

TABLE 5.7 Health Implications of Tattoos and Piercings
(*continued*)

Tattoos	Piercings
Because viral and bacterial infections, especially hepatitis B and HIV, are a concern, individuals should ensure they have received the hepatitis B immunization series and assess the tattoo especially in the early stages after application	Infection control is a key issue, especially early after the piercing insertion (HIV, hepatitis B). Mouth and nose piercings may lead to infection and dental issues that need to be assessed and managed
Removal may be costly and painful; this should be considered when deciding upon application	Piercings may close up in time, such that most piercings are more temporary than tattoos

UNINTENTIONAL INJURIES

Injuries, such as those in motor vehicle accidents and others, are the major causal factors for morbidity and mortality in the teen years. Associated factors, such as being under the influence of drugs or alcohol while driving, driving with someone under the influence, or developmental lack of appreciation of consequences, have led to the development of driving restrictions for young drivers, graduated driver's licenses, enforcement of seat belt laws, laws related to driving under the influence (DUI), strict consequences for having blood alcohol levels above 0.05 to 0.08, strict penalties for repeat DUI offenses, and other policies. Other injuries result from firearms, drowning, poisoning, fires and burns, and pedestrian accidents. Injuries may be addressed by such recommendations as the use of bicycle helmets, swimming lessons, smoke alarms, increasing use of protective equipment with sports and recreation, and educational programs about safety and injury prevention.

FOCUSED INTERVENTIONS

- Fostering a positive body image and attitude toward health is critical among teens. HCPs have a key role in ensuring that teens understand the importance of caring for their bodies.

- The four Es of fostering physical development include: Developmentally appropriate **Education** about physical development, injury prevention, nutrition, the importance of exercise, and safety; **Enactment** and **Enforcement** of policies and laws to protect the safety of teens, including those associated with injury prevention, ensuring physical activity, and nutritional patterns; and **Engineering** of product designs and systems to encourage health and safety including mechanisms for injury prevention, optimal levels of physical activity, availability of nutritious foods in key places, and safe play/recreation areas.
- Because alcohol is a major contributor to teen injuries and risk behaviors, interventions should include curtailing underage drinking, responsible drinking for older adolescents and emerging adults, and harm-reduction strategies to limit the potential consequences of overconsumption of alcohol.
- Teen-related factors, including inexperience, peer pressure, lack of maturity, increasing independence, and attraction to risk-taking behaviors, warrant that teens are aware of safety measures and are protected by adult supervision and guidance.
- Ensure that the media portray healthy, realistic, and diverse appearances and focus on other attributes besides physical appearance. HCPs may have an integral role in informing these portrayals and fostering exposure to realistic images as they develop.
- Because weight-based teasing may be one of the last sanctioned biases in society, HCPs must be vigilant to avoid prejudice and focus on health.
- Ensure same-age friends in young people who are early developers to avoid clashes or engaging in high-risk behaviors.
- Emphasis must be placed on the individuality of physical development. Each teen grows and develops at his or her own pace, manifests varying degrees of emotional and relational maturity, and presents unique issues associated with early, on-time, or late maturation.

SUGGESTED READING

Benson, L., Baer, H. J., & Kaelber, D. C. (2009). Trends in the diagnosis of overweight and obesity in children and adolescents: 1999–2007. *Pediatrics, 123,* e153–e158.

Christian, B. J. (2011). Targeting the obesity epidemic in children and adolescents: Research evidence for practice. *Journal of Pediatric Nursing, 26,* 503–506.

DiClemente, R. J., Santelli, J. S., & Crosby, R. A. (Eds.). (2009). *Adolescent health: Understanding and prevention risk behaviors.* San Francisco, CA: Jossey-Bass.

Eaton, D. K., Kann, L., Kinchen, S., Shanklin, S., Flint, K. H., Hawkins, J., . . . Wechsler, H. (2012). Youth risk behavior surveillance—United States, 2011. *MMWR, 61*(4), 1–162.

Feinstein, S. (2007). *Teaching the at-risk teenage brain.* Lanham, MD: Rowman & Littlefield.

Henderson, A., & Champlin, S. (1998). *Promoting teen health.* Thousand Oaks, CA: Sage.

Herrman, J. (2005). The teen brain as a work in progress: Implications for pediatric nurses. *Pediatric Nursing, 31,* 144–148.

McNeely, C., & Blanchard, J. (2009). *The teen years explained: A guide to healthy adolescent development.* Baltimore, MD: Johns Hopkins Bloomburg School of Public Health.

Neumark-Sztainer, D. (2005). Preventing the broad spectrum of weight-related problems: Working with parents to help teens achieve a healthy weight and a positive body image. *Journal of Nutrition Education Behavior, 37,* S133–S139.

Rome, E. S. (2012). Eating disorders in children and adolescents. *Current Problems in Pediatric Adolescent Health Care, 42,* 28–44.

Selekman, J. (2003). A new era of body decoration: What are kids doing to their bodies? *Pediatric Nursing, 29,* 77–79.

Serafini, T., Rye, B. J., & Drysdale, M. (Eds.). (2013). *Taking sides: Clashing views on adolescence.* New York, NY: McGraw-Hill.

Steinberg, L. (2008). *Adolescence.* New York, NY: McGraw-Hill.

Vallido, T., Peters, K., O'Brien, L., & Jackson, D. (2009). Sleep in adolescence: A review of issues for nursing practice. *Journal of Clinical Nursing, 18,* 1819–1826.

SUGGESTED WEBSITES

Kids Health.Org
www.kidshealth.org/teen
Child Trends
www.childtrends.org
AddHealth
www.cpc.unc.edu/projects/
addhealth
Centers for Disease Control
and Prevention
www.cdc.gov/healthyyouth
Go Ask Alice
www.goaskalice.columbia
.edu
Society for Adolescent
Medicine and Health
www.adolescenthealth.org

Healthy People
www.healthypeople.gov
Johns Hopkins School of
Public Health
www.jhsph.edu
Learn to Be Healthy
www.learntobehealthy.org/
teens
Office of Adolescent Health
www.hhs.gov/ash/oah
Teen Help.com
www.teenhelp.com

6

Intellectual Health and Risks

In the previous section, we discussed cognitive development as the teen brain went through rapid changes in structure and function. We also addressed health decision-making and how teens view health. In this chapter we continue to explore intellectual development and how selected alterations in cognitive development may impact health.

In this chapter, you will learn to:

1. Explore selected aspects of the progression of cognitive development
2. Analyze key issues, including learning disorders, autism, and attention deficit/hyperactivity disorder (ADHD), as they impact intellectual function
3. Discuss the impact of developmental disorders on teen health
4. Identify key focused interventions based upon learned concepts

COGNITIVE DEVELOPMENT

The brain follows an elaborate course of development during the teen years as individuals cross the bridge from childlike ways of thinking to adulthood. Research reveals the intricate processes that allow teens to take on the responsibilities, ideas, values, and roles of adulthood. There are three main areas of cognitive development during the teen years as noted in Table 6.1.

These cognitive processes impact teens' abilities to make sound decisions. As adults working with teens, we can do much to foster decision-making skills in teens. Like any other skill, the ability to consider all alternatives, foresee potential outcomes, and anticipate the costs and rewards of the alternatives is a product of age, practice, wisdom, and experience. Important strategies to assist teens in making sound decisions are listed in Table 6.2.

LEARNING DISORDERS, AUTISM, AND ADHD

Every teen is unique and so is the way each teen thinks, learns, and functions in our world. Selected issues may change the way teens learn, make decisions, and progress in their cognitive development. Although there are some commonalities, it is key to remember that each teen is an individual and should be recognized for his or her own abilities and needs. This section discusses learning disorders or disabilities, autism, and ADHD and how these may impact health and health practices.

Learning Disorders

This broad category describes the inability or decreased ability of an individual to understand, remember, use, or respond to information. It is generally related to a decreased ability to receive, process, or communicate information via the

TABLE 6.1 Three Tasks of Teen Cognitive Development

Tasks	Characteristics
Reasoning and decision-making skills	• Consider choices and consequences, anticipate potential alternatives, and use a logical pathway to make decisions • Increasingly capable of using rational decision-making when warranted and reserve impulsive decision-making for appropriate circumstances
Understand abstract concepts	• Formal operational thought enables comprehension of concepts that are unseen, less defined, or less concrete in nature • Provides the capacity to understand concepts such as health, pain, justice, disease, health, happiness, death, and prevention • Current theorists assert that many adults do not reach abstract reasoning, impacting how we address health education
Metacognition	• Defined as "thinking about thinking;" teens become contemplative, philosophical, and idealistic • Embrace religion and spirituality • Develop a deeper sense of empathy and use memorization strategies to enhance learning and retention • Spend a large amount of time thinking about themselves, their appearance, and their role in the world. This egocentrism or the "personal fable" perpetuates the idea that everyone is looking at them, judging them, and that every action is being watched and critiqued by others. This self-consciousness is often one of the greatest stressors during the teen years • Teens develop a strong commitment to fairness and justice. As they become more pluralistic in their learning, they are more able to see "shades of gray" and the perspectives of others

brain. The causes of learning disorders are not thoroughly understood, but may include genetic factors, environmental agents, toxins, birth trauma, brain injury, or other etiologies. Estimates of the numbers of children and teens with learning

TABLE 6.2 Strategies to Enhance Teen Decision-Making

Role model healthy decision-making

Explain decision-making to teens—we all know the frustration of "because I said so!" Encourage questioning as a way to fact find, not as questioning of authority or respect

Respect that teen decision-making may have different results than your personal deliberations

Appreciate "hot" and "cold" influences: "cold" (rational, deliberate, and conscious elements) or "hot" (emotions, passions, impulsivity, and peer pressure)

Expect respect from teens. Allow each party to respectfully express his or her thoughts and listen carefully to the thoughts of others. Teens value healthy discussion and exploration of alternatives, not to simply argue or oppose adults in their world, but as a chance to try out their newly developing skills in reasoning and communication

Ensure that teens experience the negative outcomes of poor decision-making. We sometimes try to protect teens, but living through negative repercussions offers valuable lessons

Offer frequent opportunities for decision-making

Allow teens to make mistakes. Teens need to feel empowered to make decisions by beginning with smaller ones and working their way up to more complex, life-altering decisions

Encourage teens to consider the decision-making of their peers and ruminate about the outcomes of these decisions

Encourage open sharing and free expression, and discourage any communication that makes either party feel devalued or belittled. Refrain from power struggles or winning/losing

Help teens reason through their thoughts and feelings. Emotions like anger, frustration, jealousy, disappointment, and sadness are often difficult to differentiate and may have varying impacts on the decision-making process. Help teens see how these emotions may alter their options and the influence they exert on rational decision-making

Offer the immediate and long-term consequences of actions as teens consider their options. Teens' thoughts often focus on the "here and now." Providing longer-term ideas about the costs and rewards of an action may assist in the teen's development of future-oriented thinking

(continued)

TABLE 6.2 Strategies to Enhance Teen Decision-Making (continued)	
Offer respect for the teens' choices, even if not in agreement, as teens consider their options. Rather than criticizing the teens' conclusions, explore the potential outcomes of their choices and how they may look in the future. Assist teens to consider multiple perspectives and when there is "more than one right answer"	The teen years may be characterized by "adolescent hypocrisy" in which teens know and talk about one behavior and yet do not act in a similar manner. The cognitive development during the teen years paves the way for this behavior and adults should be aware of such behaviors in middle school and as they subside during the high school years
Consider the "immediate and certain" versus the "delayed and uncertain" consequences associated with decision-making	Ask teens to think through in role play or "what if" scenarios; explaining rationales may be a valuable way to understand reasoning

disorders are highly variable. Learning disorders may be specific or general.

- Specific learning disorders may:
  - Impact one or more areas of intellectual functioning but intelligence is not impaired
  - See Table 6.3 for types of specific learning disorders
- Generalized learning disorders may:
  - Impact all intellectual functions
  - Be significant enough to lead to a developmental delay
  - Include physical or motor involvement
  - Include behavioral disorders

These learning differences are best managed in a supportive academic environment that includes family education and counseling, individualized care and planning, and an understanding of the unique characteristics of each learner. Resources indicate that learning disorders may persist throughout adulthood and recommend training programs

TABLE 6.3 Common Specific Learning Disorders

Type	Description
Dyslexia	Impaired ability to read or write; difficulties with reading, writing, organizing thoughts, and processing sequences
Dysgraphia	An inability to write and spell, hampered fine motor and idea processing skills
Auditory processing disorder	Difficulty distinguishing among sounds and with language
Visual processing disorder	Difficult with reading and interpreting visual stimuli
Dyscalculia	Difficulty learning mathematical principles and performing calculations
Amusia	Inability to recognize musical notes and rhythms or to replicate tunes or sounds
Dyspraxia/apraxia	Inability to work with objects in space, to move or manipulate objects, or to understand spatial relationships; may also include diminished speech and ability to articulate words
Specific language impairment	Difficulty in receptive and expressive language function despite adequate hearing and motor function

that foster coping skills and personal control such that adults are able to adapt and flourish as they encounter learning issues during the adult years. Mainstreaming, in which learners of all levels are taught in the same classroom and resources are available to meet the needs of individuals, has become a common practice in today's educational world. Not only is mainstreaming for children with learning disorders mandated by federal law, but it also provides academic challenge, provides exposure to social and interpersonal relationships, reduces stigma, and encourages helpfulness and social integration. Another population to consider is the overlap of children and teens with learning disorders attempting to learn English as a second language. English-language learners with learning disorders, anticipated to comprise 25% of students by 2020, will require significant resources in order to succeed in school and the work world.

FAST FACTS in a NUTSHELL

Schoolchildren in the United States with and without identified learning disorders require additional support and services; for example:

27% of students are below grade level for reading
26% of students are below grade level for writing
32% of students with learning disorders drop out of school (compared with 10% of students without learning disorders)
11% of students with learning disorders attend college (compared with 53% of students without learning disorders)

Autism

Autism is a rare spectrum of disorders with various forms and manifestations. The symptoms of autism usually begin before the age of 3 years and include problems with social reciprocity, language or communication difficulties, self-destructive behavior, unusual interests and behaviors, and restriction in interests or repetitive behaviors. Individuals with autism may experience these signs and symptoms in varying degrees, with the inability to understand the mental processes of others and reflect on one's own thoughts serving as the core of the condition. This lack of processing, inherent in autism, is described as the inability to engage the "Theory of the Mind" (the ability to understand that others hold different thoughts and beliefs and that these may impact the outcomes of a situation). Types of autism are given in Table 6.4.

TABLE 6.4 Types of Autism

Type	Description
Classic or autistic disorder	Includes classic symptoms of impaired social skills, poor communication, and repetitive behaviors. The individual may: avoid eye and physical contact, fail to respond to name or being spoken to, rock or engage in continuous movements, be disturbed by change, have delayed speech with abnormal tone, develop specific routines, be sensitive to sensory signals, have learning difficulties, and may have high level of abilities in one area
Savant syndrome	Exceptional abilities in one area of learning, including math, design, or music
Asperger's syndrome	Similar to classic autism but less severe, have average or above-average intelligence, may have a narrow range of interests, may have impaired social skills, and may be inflexible in behaviors and routines
Rett syndrome	A rare form of autism impacting females wherein the child develops normally until about 1 or 2 years of age, then development regresses and autistic behaviors appear
Childhood disintegrative disorder	A rare form of autism impacting males wherein the child develops normally until about 3 or 4 years of age, then development regresses and autistic behaviors appear

There is no cure for autism. Treatment is focused on behavioral therapy, supportive academic stimulation to the potential of the individual, and family education and counseling.

ADHD

ADHD is one of the most common behavioral conditions of childhood. Sources indicate that between 4% to 5% and 4% to 12% (9% of males and 3% of females) of young people are diagnosed with ADHD. Some believe that this number will increase as we become increasingly technology based, value multitasking, reinforce immediate gratification, and are less reliant on physical work and activity in our daily lives. Most individuals are usually diagnosed in their school-age years and early diagnosis ensures the optimal opportunity for the child and family to adjust to the diagnosis. As children approach adolescence and the school workload becomes more taxing, requiring increased focus and attentiveness, there is also an increase in the number of teens diagnosed with ADHD. Diagnosis of ADHD during adolescence may be a challenge since it may be difficult to differentiate "normal" teen behaviors and those associated with ADHD. Some believe that children "outgrow" ADHD but the symptoms may continue into the teen and adult years.

FAST FACTS in a NUTSHELL

Eighty percent of all those diagnosed with ADHD as children experience symptoms as teens; 60% of those with symptoms as teens experience ADHD symptoms as adults.

ADHD is thought to have genetic, environmental/toxic, and organic (such as birth trauma) causation. It appears that there are low dopamine levels related to ADHD; therefore, medications that increase dopamine are effective in managing symptoms. The types of ADHD are noted in Table 6.5.

TABLE 6.5 Types of ADHD

Type	Characteristics
Inattentive	Short attention span, poor concentration, difficulty with change, inability to follow instructions, distractibility, inability to focus
Hyperactive/ impulsive	Fidgeting, acting without thinking, excessive talking, interrupting others, short temper or emotional lability, recklessness
Combined	Symptoms of both types

6. INTELLECTUAL HEALTH AND RISKS

ADHD, and its impact on brain executive functions, may lead to low self-esteem in individuals, impact their social and family lives, and hamper academic performance. ADHD is associated with grade retention, difficulties with graduation, and poorer performance on standardized tests. ADHD has a large number of comorbidities, including depression, anxiety, conduct disorders, oppositional disorders, and bipolar disorder. For example, between 20% and 60% of teens with ADHD also have learning disorders.

Some teens with ADHD may hyperfocus or be intensely attentive to one activity. They also may have a poor sense of time and sequencing of events. This may lead to short-sighted actions without regard for future implications of behavior. As with most teens, education of teens with ADHD about prevention should focus on immediate and relevant consequences of actions. Nonetheless, during the teen years, the impulsivity and poor anger control associated with ADHD may lead to participation in high-risk behaviors, including abuse of drugs, tobacco, and alcohol; risky sexual activity; gambling; eating disorders; the potential for motor vehicle accidents; and delinquency. Changes in self-image and frustration may lead to self-medication with drugs and alcohol. Recent research indicated that male youth with ADHD were twice as likely to be arrested as young men without ADHD.

FAST FACTS in a NUTSHELL

Teens who take stimulants or other pharmacologic treatments for ADHD cut their risk for using substances by two thirds and have a reduced likelihood to become addicted to substances.

Smoking has a calming effect on some people with ADHD and increases attentiveness and inhibitory control (this is not an endorsement for smoking but may indicate nicotine treatment as an area for future research!).

Management of ADHD is based on targeted symptoms, and treatment is dual focused, including behavioral therapy and medications. Family and individual education and counseling including key stakeholders in the child's world such as teachers and caregivers is the first line of treatment. If symptoms continue, medications may be added. In fact, behavioral treatments may be more effective after medications are initiated and as the child demonstrates an increased ability to attend to, focus, and control his or her own behavior. Stimulant medications, such as methylphenidate (Ritalin), block dopamine binding sites, allowing for more free dopamine to remain in the system. Other nonstimulant agents are also effective in managing the symptoms of ADHD.

Ongoing education and teaching about ADHD are critical. Researchers noted that there are significant misunderstandings about ADHD, such as the role of sugar in ADHD symptomatology. Health care providers (HCPs) may do much to clarify these misconceptions. It is estimated that 10% of all children have been prescribed ADHD medications, leading some to believe that the medication is overused. Additional concerns exist about drug diversion and illicit abuse of Ritalin and other stimulants by adolescents and college students to stay awake to work and study.

THE IMPACT OF DEVELOPMENTAL DISORDERS ON HEALTH

The preceding information was not an exhaustive discussion of developmental disorders but was meant to stimulate you to consider how teens with these conditions may experience health and what we, as HCPs, need to do to promote their health and well-being. Several factors jeopardize a teen's health when he or she is impacted by a developmental disorder:

- Health literacy is a concern for most people as the health care world is difficult to navigate. Teens and those with special needs may require increased assistance to understand care and their personal role in maintaining health.

- Several of the disorders discussed in this chapter are related to serious comorbidities and other problems. Knowledge of these is important such that HCPs may screen and educate teens accordingly.
- Characteristics of teen brain development, including sensation-seeking, response to peer pressure, enthusiasm, creativity, present orientation, the need for immediate relevance, the growing ability to control impulses, and the sensitivity to rewards rather than punishment, impact how teens make decisions, their involvement in high-risk behaviors, and their health status.
- Key roles of HCPs are advocating for teens, assisting families and teens to self-advocate, and connecting those without resources or family support to appropriate agencies.
- Developmental disorders may be associated with high-risk behaviors and this will amplify the stress experienced by teens and families. Support and counseling may optimize their ability to cope with these stressors.

Some basic principles include:

- Use developmental age, not chronological age, to determine teens' abilities, their personal capacity for learning, and their role in self-care. Do not make the assumption that teens with developmental delay are regressed in all areas. For example, teens with developmental delay often experience age-appropriate sexual desires and require education and access to services to ensure safe sexual behavior.
- Although it is important to screen for diagnosed developmental disorders, our society is also quick to label individuals. We need to balance identification of needs with ways to limit the stigma associated with such labels in teens' schools, homes, health care settings, and communities.

- Each teen has his or her own potential and talents. Our plans of care need to focus on these unique talents.
- Teens often do not like to be singled out and, therefore, may be resistant to individualized instructional support or health care. We need to balance confidentiality with the need for services.
- Adolescents treasure control of their lives—we can foster positive results and relationships by allowing teens, while attending to their developmental abilities, to retain control and have a say in their own health care.
- Many individuals with developmental disorders are entitled by federal and other legislation to accommodations. Students in schools have Individual Health Plans (IHPs) and Individual Educational Plans (IEPs) to ensure care specific to the needs of these children.
- Those with developmental disorders are disproportionately represented among those living in poverty. This places individuals at risk for significant health disparities and calls upon HCPs for even stronger advocacy efforts.

FOCUSED INTERVENTIONS

- Decision-making is a critical skill in the developing teen. Ongoing attention to fostering this ability in all teens, regardless of level of cognitive function, assists teens to mature to their greatest personal potential. As teens mature and their health decision-making reflects an understanding of personal responsibility for health, teens will be better able to understand the power of prevention.
- As teens progress in development, their idealism and enthusiasm gives them the energy to dedicate huge efforts toward "causes." This development of selflessness should be encouraged as teens begin to appreciate the needs of others and the value of providing services to their peers, families, or others.

- Use open-ended questions to stimulate discussions with teens. Using the word "why" could make the teen feel defensive or needing to justify his or her conclusions.
- Be careful to avoid public embarrassment of teens. This is true for any age but teens may have a difficult time trusting an adult who has made them feel less worthy in front of their peers and others.
- Help teens learn to recognize and identify their emotions and those of others. Teens may confuse their personal feelings, misinterpreting disappointment, embarrassment, or frustration for anger. One way to do this is to develop an emotions library. In this exercise, teens come up with a list of as many emotions as they can think of and keep the list with them. When they encounter a difficult decision, they use the list to identify the emotions they are feeling about the situation, the decision, and its outcomes. By clarifying the emotion, teens may be better able to confront the decision while attending to the concurrent emotions.
- As teens age, they accrue greater numbers of past experiences upon which to draw when considering resolution or alternatives in decision-making. Help teens see the value of this learning and to remember past events that may help inform the current decision.

SUGGESTED READING

Beren, M. (2002). ADHD in adolescence: Will you know it when you see it? *Contemporary Pediatrics, 19*(4), 124–143.

Bussing, R., Zima, B. T., Mason, D. M., Meyer, J. M., White, M. D., & Garvan, C. W. (2012). ADHD knowledge, perceptions, and information sources: Perspectives from a community sample of adolescents and their parents. *Journal of Adolescent Health, 51*, 593–600.

Byrnes, J. P. (2002). The development of decision-making. *Journal of Adolescent Health, 31*, 208–215.

Carter, R. (2009). *The human brain book.* New York, NY: DK.

Childress, A. C., & Berry, S. A. (2012). Pharmacotherapy of ADHD in adolescents. *Drugs, 72*(3), 309–325.

DiClemente, R. J., Santelli, J. S., & Crosby, R. A. (Eds.). (2009). *Adolescent health: Understanding and prevention risk behaviors.* San Francisco, CA: Jossey-Bass.

Feinstein, S. (2007). *Teaching the at-risk teenage brain.* Lanham, MD: Rowman & Littlefield.

Firth, N., Frydenberg, E., & Greaves, D. (2008). Perceived control and adaptive coping: Program for adolescent student who have learning disabilities. *Learning Disability Quarterly, 31,* 151–164.

Herrman, J. (2005). The teen brain as a work in progress: Implications for pediatric nurses. *Pediatric Nursing, 31,* 144–148.

Lauer-Bradbury, C. (2012). The treatment of ADHD in children and young people. *British Journal of School Nursing, 7*(2), 71–75.

McNeely, C., & Blanchard, J. (2009). *The teen years explained: A guide to healthy adolescent development.* Baltimore, MD: Johns Hopkins Bloomburg School of Public Health.

National Joint Committee on Learning Disabilities. (2008). Adolescent literacy and older students with learning disabilities. *Learning Disability Quarterly, 31,* 211–218.

Robinson, R. (2004). It's a brain thing: Teens, ADHD, and binge drinking. *Neurology Today, 4*(3), 16–17.

Schaefer, A., Collette, F., Philippot, P., van der Linden, M., Laureys, S., Delfiore, G., . . . Salmon, E. (2003). Neural correlates of "hot" and "cold" emotional processing: A multilevel approach to the functional anatomy of emotion. *NeuroImage, 18,* 938–949.

Steinberg, L. (2008). *Adolescence.* New York, NY: McGraw-Hill.

Sutherland, P. (1999). The application of Piagetian and neo-Piagetian ideas to further and higher education. *International Journal of Lifelong Education, 18,* 286–295.

Sweeney, M. S. (2009). *Brain: The complete mind, how it develops, how it works, and how to keep it sharp.* Washington, DC: National Geographic.

SUGGESTED WEBSITES

Kids Health.Org
www.kidshealth.org/teen

Advocates for Youth
www.advocatesforyouth.org

Child Trends
www.childtrends.org

The Search Institute
www.search-institute.org

The Bureau For At-Risk Youth
www.at-risk.com

Go Ask Alice
www.goaskalice.columbia.edu

Society for Adolescent
   Medicine and Health
   www.adolescenthealth.org
Healthy People
   www.healthypeople.gov

Johns Hopkins School of
   Public Health
   www.jhsph.edu
Office of Adolescent Health
   www.hhs.gov/ash/oah

7

Emotional Health and Risks

The teen years are a time of growth, fun, and happiness, but are also a time of emotional turbulence, searching, and ambivalence. Every teen endeavors to establish his or her identity or "comfortable place" in the world. Teens reflect on peers' identities and build on the foundation of their family and the environment to develop a sense of self that helps them handle the challenges of adulthood. Mental health issues may range from moderate stress in response to daily life demands to total affliction. It is estimated that 20% to 50% of all teens experience some level of mental health issues and, of those, about 60% to 90% do not receive treatment. Undiagnosed and untreated mental health conditions may lead to violence, homelessness, poverty, abuse, delinquency, and substance abuse. Health care providers (HCPs) should be aware of such mental health issues and of their impact on teen health as another component of holistic care.

In this chapter, you will learn to:

1. Describe the process of identity formation during the teen years
2. Analyze the role of stress in mental health
3. Explain how depression, anxiety, suicide, self-cutting, and the use of substances influence teen health
4. Identify key focused interventions based upon learned concepts

IDENTITY FORMATION AND MENTAL HEALTH

Developing a personal identity and sense of self is one of the critical tasks of the teen years. How teens perceive themselves may change with the day, context, or mood. The identity development process is one of experimentation, reinforcement, and exploration. Personal identity includes self-concept, or what one thinks or believes about oneself, and self-esteem. Self-esteem is how one feels emotionally about oneself and may be affected by the approval of others. For example, body image is a prominent component of self-esteem, is based on feelings about one's body and appearance, and may be subject to the approval of others. For most teens this process is most intense during the middle school years and stabilizes during the later adolescent years—but we continue to shape our identity throughout our lives. Many contend that positive self-concept and self-esteem are protective factors against engagement in high-risk behaviors. The tasks associated with teen development of an identity are shown in Table 7.1.

Teens often perseverate on their weaknesses or perceived areas of deficiency rather than thoroughly examining their personal assets. Critics contend that today's society rewards a limited scope of success, requiring all teens to be academically gifted, skilled in athletics, and socially adept. It may be helpful to allow teens to consider their strengths based on the theory of multiple intelligences. Gardner introduced the need to recognize and appreciate the existence of multiple intelligences with which individuals process the world around them. In this model, humans function from a framework of $8\frac{1}{2}$ intelligences (Table 7.2).

TABLE 7.1 Teen Identity Development

Stage	Description
Creating a sense of independence	Achieving physical and psychological autonomy from parents and family, supported by parental guidance and the provision of boundaries
Developing a sense of mastery	Through exploring new skills, teens appraise their strengths and weaknesses and establish areas of competence. This is both unconscious and conscious. Cultivating talents decreases the propensity for depression and increases coping abilities
Establishing social place or social status	Teens determine where they stand in a group and reflect on their need for belonging and "fitting in"
Achieving intimacy	Relationships with parents, friends, and intimate partners are characterized by love, trust, and honesty
Understanding personal sexual identity	Teens think about, question, reflect on, or act on sexual orientation, gender orientation, and aspects of personal sexuality

TABLE 7.2 Gardner's 8½ Intelligences

Verbal/linguistic

Logical/mathematical

Visual/spatial

Body/kinesthetic

Musical

Naturalist

Interpersonal

Intrapersonal

Existentialist/spiritual (½)

Self-analysis of these multiple intelligences is an important part of personal growth. Allowing teens to assess their strengths in these areas helps enhance their sense of mastery, provides them with goals for future efforts, and may inform their life goals as they consider educational and career routes that build on their innate abilities.

STRESS

Stress is a physiological response to stimuli and is necessary for survival. It is stress that makes us take the next breath, stay alert, eat a meal, be attentive, study for a test, walk a little faster, and motivates us to act and function in daily life. In mild to moderate levels, stress is a positive part of human nature. When stress levels exceed the ability to cope, the individual may experience changes in mood, ability to function, and personal feelings of well-being. Table 7.3 illustrates the potential signs of stress overload.

The release of norepinephrine, a neurotransmitter, and cortisol, known as the stress hormone, enhances energy and increases coping skills in order to reduce stress levels. If allowed to increase to an unacceptable level, stressors may overwhelm, incapacitate, and damage an individual. High cortisol levels increase heart rate and blood pressure, diminish immune system function, deplete body reserves, result in fatigue and low levels of energy, and may sustain these negative effects long after exposure to the stress. Teens may have unique responses to stress (Table 7.4).

The teenage years are times of stress. Establishing a personal identity, achieving independence, dealing with peer pressure, and other stimuli breed stress in teens. Studies have indicated that the major stressors in teens' lives differ from those of other individuals, as cited in Table 7.5. Low-income teens who are living in poverty, in threatening neighborhoods, and with less stable families may be at risk for increased stress.

TABLE 7.3 Signs of Stress Overload

Chronic headaches	Withdrawal	Nervousness
Stomachaches	Irritability	Changes in eating habits
Frequent, vague symptoms	Crying	Changes in sleeping habits
Fatigue	Difficulty concentrating	Mood variability

TABLE 7.4 Teens' Unique Responses to Stress

Teens take longer to recover from stress	Teens sustain more significant vital sign changes
Teens have higher cortisol release in responses to stress	Teens have more drastic physiological responses to stress
High levels of progesterone in teen girls prolong the stress response	Teens are especially vulnerable to experiencing and suffering from the stress response
Without a developed prefrontal cortex, teens are less able to use coping strategies	Teens experiencing trauma may appear to be coping well but lack the ability to deal with additional stressors
Chronic stress is associated with a smaller hippocampus, decreasing the capacity for memory and learning	Reduced frontal lobe function allows the amygdala to dominate teens' reactions, including fear, anger, rage, and other primitive reactions

TABLE 7.5 Major Stressors as Ranked by Teens

School, school demands, school performance, and impact on life goals	Money, work, and financial responsibilities
Parents and family conflict/home life	Dress, clothes, and current styles
Dating and relationships	Puberty/gender/sexual orientation
Friends and peer pressure	Appearance/pressure for body perfection
Moving, relocation, and tenuous home situations	Parental marital discord and divorce
Establishing identity	The future

Although our society considers stress as a negative, we must learn to keep positive stressors at an optimal level, learn to recognize and manage stress that is growing to an uncontrolled level, and use coping strategies when stress is about to cause negative effects. Addressing stress immediately and realistically, realizing the continuous nature

TABLE 7.6 Stress Management Strategies

Talk about your problems	Take deep breaths
Give up on perfection	Take a walk in a comfortable place
Use progressive muscle tension and relaxation	Take a minute to "roll your neck" and stretch out tight upper back muscles
Assemble and use a list of affirmations about your strengths	Use imagery and imagine places and events that are happy and stress free
Pray or recite consoling phrases	Sing or hum a favorite or comforting song
Engage in exercise (work out, yoga, Pilates, run, lift weights, bike ride, walk fast, stretch, etc.)	Explore the "worst case" scenario, consider whether that situation is realistic and the likelihood of that scenario actually occurring
Use journaling, drama, art, and other methods of expression	Let go of the situation and allow yourself to move on
Plan projects in manageable pieces	Picture how you will work, feel, and be after the stressor is over

of stress, and engaging in stress management strategies are important parts of teen development and our teaching (Table 7.6).

MENTAL HEALTH ISSUES: DEPRESSION, ANXIETY, AND SUICIDE

The teen years themselves are characterized by the search for identity, mood swings, emotional upheaval, exaggerated responses to difficult situations, and ongoing stress. Lower levels of serotonin in teens may be related to their potential for negative moods. At times it is difficult to differentiate "normal teen behavior" and mental health issues requiring intervention. Mental health issues range from mild to severe. When issues impact functioning at school, home, in relationships, or when there is a significant change in behavior or habits, treatment may be needed. Some mental health

One in five teens has a diagnosable mental health disorder.

More than one half of all mental health disorders begin by age 14; three quarters by age 24.

More than one in four teens report having at least mild symptoms of depression.

Thirty-six percent of teen women and 22% of teen men reported feeling sad or hopeless for 2 weeks in the previous year (average 29%).

Some sources indicate that twice the females as males experience depression.

disorders diagnosed during childhood may diminish as teens reach adulthood, while others may persist. The availability of a supportive, dependable, and caring adult is very valuable as teens deal with difficult times.

Depression

Depression is a significant issue among teens, and those working with teens should be familiar with the signs of depression and the resources in their area to provide treatment. Depression has many causes and, for most individuals, the etiology remains multifactorial. Genetic, experiential, environmental, and traumatic events may spur depression. Other associated factors include stressful life events, being of racial and ethnic minorities, and histories of physical or sexual abuse. The neurotransmitter serotonin is responsible for mood stabilization and is thought to provide feelings of contentment and satisfaction. Deficiencies in serotonin in some individuals may cause depressive symptoms. This led to the success of the medication class selective serotonin reuptake inhibitors. This popular class of medications allows for an increased level of serotonin and is thought to elevate

TABLE 7.7 Signs of Depression in Teens

Irritability	Physical complaints (stomachache or headache)
Anger	School absence or decreased performance
Social withdrawal	Low energy
Change in appetite or sleep habits	Feeling overwhelmed
Feeling sad or hopeless	Intention of suicide
Crying	History of running away
Decreased interest or pleasure (anhedonia)	Decreased concentration
Fatigue	Changes in relationships

moods in those with minor and major depressive disorders. Depression is characterized by a variety of manifestations as presented in Table 7.7.

Management of depression requires assessment and monitoring by those qualified to provide treatment that is adapted for the unique needs of teens. Cognitive behavioral therapy, which assists teens to verbalize their concerns, reframe sad thoughts and perceptions, modify negative thoughts, and anticipate positive changes in their lives, is now a cornerstone of treatment. Family therapy, interpersonal therapy, education, exercise programs, medication with antidepressants, and trauma-informed care are also important adjuncts to care.

Anxiety

If stress can be traced to specific causative factors, then anxiety is worry and anguish that is often without an identifiable origin or when symptoms are significant enough to impair function. Anxiety disorders are major problems in teens and may compound teen stressors leading to difficulties in coping with the demands of day-to-day life. About 10% of teens suffer from anxiety in the United States today. Anxiety is actually a cluster of disorders. Anxiety disorders also have a high level of comorbidity with depression. Bullying, living in unsafe or traumatic environments, poverty, and chronic stress have been associated with the development of anxiety disorders. Like other mental health issues, anxiety has genetic, environmental, and experiential causative elements and is thought to be related to decreased levels of serotonin. Anxiety disorders are described in Table 7.8.

Treatment for anxiety includes counseling, education about coping and stress management strategies, and medications. The anxiolytics (drugs used to treat anxiety) must be monitored carefully because many cause physical and emotional dependence and tolerance. The alleviation or reduction of the stressful or traumatic circumstances causing the anxiety is also essential in comprehensively managing the teen with anxiety. As with depression, counseling, service coordination, medications, and therapy work together to assist teens and their families and friends in managing anxiety disorders.

TABLE 7.8 Anxiety Disorders

Disorder	Description
Obsessive compulsive disorder	Recurrent and persistent thoughts that are unwanted; repetitive behaviors or rituals
Social anxiety disorder	Disturbance related to social experiences and events
Posttraumatic stress disorder	Flashbacks, bad dreams, emotional numbness, and intense worry or guilt after a dangerous or frightening event
Phobias	Intense fears of things or circumstances that pose little or no actual danger
Panic attacks	Physical symptoms associated with a disturbing event (including testing, athletic events, public speaking, or others)

Suicide

In recent years, suicide has been either the second- or third-most common cause of death among teenagers. Any death of a teen is difficult but a suicide may be especially tragic.

There may be signs that an individual is contemplating suicide. Any expression of the desire to hurt or kill oneself should be taken seriously and reported to appropriate resources (Table 7.9).

FAST FACTS in a NUTSHELL

At the time of an attempted or completed suicide:

- 90% of teens were diagnosed with a mental disorder.
- 60% were suffering from depression at the time of death.

In the United States, 6.3% of teens attempted suicide in the past year.

- Young women tend to attempt suicide more than young men.
- Young men are more successful at suicide attempts (related to the accessibility and lethality of guns).

TABLE 7.9 Potential Signs of Suicide

Withdrawal	Change in eating, sleeping, and hygiene habits
Talking about leaving	A plan for suicide
A significant loss	Talking about suicide in school and with peers
Preoccupation with suicide, death, and morbid topics	Giving away personal objects of importance
Decreased level of concentration	Suicidal ideations
Talking about future relief from pain	A sudden appearance of elation or relief

Maintaining teen safety is paramount and adults working with teens need to understand, and share with teens, the concept of conditional confidentiality. Communication with teens will be kept confidential unless teens express the desire to hurt themselves or others. Most teens report some level of ambivalence about their plan for suicide. Anyone interfacing with teens should be vigilant for those at risk for suicide or manifesting potential indications of suicide. Even off-hand references to self-harm or the world without them should be followed up and the teens should be assessed and supported. There is some concern about "copycat" suicide practices causing some communities to be extra watchful for suicide among teens and to implement prevention practices.

The role of HCPs as mandatory reporters ensures that teens expressing suicidal ideations or believed to be at risk for self-harm are kept safe and referred for intensive treatment. If the teen is in an area where immediate treatment is delayed, the HCP should ensure that the teen is monitored at all times, the environment is cleared of any potentially harmful objects, and the individual is supported and cared for until help arrives. It is important to directly confront someone believed to be contemplating suicide. Table 7.10 includes selected questions to ask.

TABLE 7.10 Questions to Assess Suicide Risk

Tell me about difficulties in your life right how.

Has anyone ever hurt you? Have you ever been abused?

Do you know anyone who has ever wanted to hurt himself or herself or anyone who has committed suicide?

Have you ever wished you were dead?

Have you ever felt so unhappy you thought about killing yourself?

Do you want to hurt or kill yourself now?

Have you ever tried to hurt or kill yourself in the past?

Do you have a plan to harm yourself?

Do you have access to a weapon or means to harm yourself?

Although teens with depression, teens undergoing treatment with antidepressant medications, and teens experiencing trauma and loss should be assessed carefully for the potential for suicide, any teen may be at risk at times of stress or crisis. Remembering the fragility of teens and the need for ongoing development of coping skills to deal with stress are important in suicide prevention. Resources report the importance and effectiveness of suicide prevention education programs in schools.

SELF-CUTTING

Self-cutting or "cutting" is a relatively common and misunderstood practice among teens and young adults. Cutting may happen at any age, in any race or socioeconomic status, and in both genders, and it is most common among young women. It is estimated that more than 2 million people engage in self-harm practices each year. Knives and sharp instruments are most commonly used in cutting, although other forms of self-harm occur. Though some think that cutting is done as an expression of self-hate or a desire to hurt or kill oneself, cutting is actually a coping mechanism to relieve tension in response to significant stress, anxiety, or lack of control. Most "cutters" know and avoid major vessels that would lead to bleeding and instead pick surfaces of the skin such as the abdomen or forearm. According to experts, the individual feels significant inner pain and cutting allows for the physical manifestation or release of the inner feelings. It is thought that cutting releases endorphins, or hormones of elation, and dopamine. The liberation of these chemicals as a result of the cutting episode provides some explanation for the addictive qualities of cutting. Others voice the "numbness" they feel to the emotional trauma they perceive in their lives. The act of using a knife or other tool to cut their skin provides them with the ability to feel "something" and mourn their loss or feel sadness. Some maintain that cutting is part of a self-destructive pattern that coincides with guilt or self-blame.

Cutting is often detected by visualizing the cuts, noting clothes inappropriate for the weather, or divulging of the practices by the individual. Cutting may also be associated with depression or anorexia, but the exact origin of this behavior is unknown. Whatever the cause, cutting is a problem that requires professional intervention. Young people who are aware of peers' cutting behaviors should be instructed to tell an adult about the behavior. Individuals should be referred to counseling, and therapy is often indicated for the teen and the family. Even with treatment, 40% to 60% of those treated for cutting continue to do so after formal therapy is over.

SUBSTANCE USE AND ABUSE: ALCOHOL, DRUGS, AND TOBACCO

Substance use is thought by selected authorities to be an experimental, perhaps normative, part of the teenage experience. For some teens, this use is excessive and leads to myriad sequelae. Substance use often includes mental health comorbidities. Teens are especially vulnerable to the impact of drugs, alcohol, and tobacco. Not only is adolescence a time for risk-taking, experimentation, peer pressure, and self-medication for stress and mood changes, but the teen brain is extra sensitive to the addictive qualities of these substances and is resistant to treatment or cessation. Alcohol and drug use releases dopamine into the system. This dopamine stimulates the reward system, allowing the teen to feel pleasure and stimulating the desire for more. Drugs like cocaine block the dopamine receptors, allowing more free-floating, active dopamine. The dopamine decreases impulse control, makes teens less sensitive to the satisfaction with rewards, reduces executive functioning skills, and may cause exaggerated emotional responses. Unfortunately, habitual drug use reduces the body's innate ability to activate dopamine and feel rewards from daily stimuli. The body seeks out newer and increasingly novel stimuli to feel pleasure. More exposure to the substance makes it harder and harder for the teen to feel a natural pleasure response. This causes teens to seek out more intense and increasingly powerful agents to feel good.

Research tells us that teens who partake in binge drinking in the early teen years are at increased risk for addiction later in life. When exposed to drugs, alcohol, and tobacco during the pruning process, the brain is highly susceptible to later addiction and difficulties in cessation. Generally, if adults drink too much alcohol, they become tired and eventually pass out. Teens, in contrast, do not experience these symptoms until much later and can drink much more at one time. Because teens do not react the same way as adults to large amounts of alcohol, teens are at risk for both overindulgence and the potential for alcohol poisoning. Potential indicators of substance use are included in Table 7.11.

Frequent drinking of alcohol, binge drinking, alcohol addiction, and substance use are dangerous for the developing brain. Research revealed that teens with drinking problems have a smaller hippocampus and demonstrate both short- and long-term memory loss as a result of drinking. In addition, impairment to the prefrontal cortex results in chronic issues with impulse control, aggression, and poor decision-making. The delayed connections of the limbic system with the prefrontal cortex may lead to misinterpretation of emotional stimuli. Girls are thought to be more susceptible to the negative effects of alcohol on brain activity; therefore, these changes in brain structure and function may be even more devastating for girls. Alcoholism and some substance use are thought to have genetic, environmental, and experiential origins.

TABLE 7.11 Signs of Potential Substance Use or Abuse

Mood changes	Friends with addiction issues
Loss or change of friends	Hangovers
Defensiveness	Fatigue
Dishonesty with peers and parents about alcohol	Withdrawal from activities or meeting obligations
Changes in friends or social life	Memory loss

- The average age of initial use of alcohol is 13 to 14 years of age.
- 75% percent of teens have used substances, alcohol, or cigarettes (by high school graduation, this climbs to 88%), including:
  - 72% of teens used alcohol
  - 46% used cigarettes
  - 37% used marijuana
  - 65% used more than one substance
- ½ of teens live with adults who have problematic substance abuse patterns.
- ⅓ of all adolescents may be described as having personal problematic substance abuse.
- Youth who drink before age 15 are four times more likely to develop alcohol dependency as those who start later.
- 50% percent of fatal motor vehicle accidents in 15- to 24-year-olds are related to alcohol.
- 40% of DUI arrests are in individuals less than 24 years of age.

Education about alcohol and the hazards of drinking have been moderately effective in reducing alcohol consumption among teens, but pockets of teens still have high rates of use. Designated driver policies, stiff penalties for driving under the influence, and strong enforcement of laws requiring identification for purchase have facilitated this reduction. Alcohol-related motor vehicle accidents remain a leading cause of morbidity and mortality among teens and warrant ongoing efforts in this area.

Although underage drinking should not be encouraged, many individuals and cultures endorse the "forbidden fruit" philosophy about drinking. Families and others espouse that drinking small amounts of alcohol as part of religious holidays, family events and celebrations, or as part of traditional meals or customs allows teens to see alcohol drinking in a "normalized" light wherein personal responsibility and moderation prevail.

The drug problem in the United States has changed such that marijuana, heroin, cocaine, and diverted prescription drugs (pain relievers, tranquilizers, sedatives, and stimulants) are the agents of most significant concern. Today's stronger concentrations of marijuana than in previous decades raise concerns about current use. Less common drugs such as amphetamines, inhalants, and ecstasy are still used and warrant ongoing prevention efforts.

FAST FACTS in a NUTSHELL

- Two million teens use inhalants each year.
- Inhalants are the drug of choice for 13- and 14-year-olds.
- 3.4% of 12-year-olds and 4.8% of 13-year-olds report to have used inhalants.
- Inhalants include adhesives, aerosols, solvents, food sprays, and bottled gases.

There is evidence that the teen brain is especially sensitive to the addictive qualities of nicotine. About 35% of teens report daily smoking of tobacco related to peer pressure, stress, addiction, and parental role modeling. In addition to being the leading preventable cause of death, smokers who begin before 21 years of age may find it the hardest to quit. Concern has been expressed over advertisers targeting teens with glamorized images of smokers and smoking based on the knowledge that, for teens, as few as several cigarettes or smoking for a short time has been shown to make the body crave nicotine. Teens of mothers who smoked during pregnancy are the most vulnerable to dependence because of prenatal exposure and sensitivity to nicotine.

In addition to the well-known impacts of smoking on respiratory and cardiovascular functions, smoking may affect memory and learning and has been correlated with depression and life-threatening cardiac dysrhythmias. Interventions that are related to the long-term impact of smoking such as lung disease or other negative consequences are relatively ineffective with teens. Instead, more policy-oriented strategies including raising the price of cigarettes, limiting smoking areas, and requiring identification to purchase cigarettes appear more effective in reducing teen smoking rates. Education and prevention strategies that focus on the immediate physical, sports, and appearance aspects of smoking may be critical in teen-focused initiatives. Controversy exists over the use of nicotine replacement therapy for teens as a means to promote smoking cessation.

FOCUSED INTERVENTIONS

- Capitalize on the positive elements of peer support and peer pressure, including peer mentors and peer educators. Encourage teens to identify, support, and refer friends who are experiencing mental health issues, substance use problems, or emotional difficulties.
- Attend to characteristics of teen development in prevention education, including risk-taking, consequences that are immediate and relevant, peer pressure, and self-medication.
- Prevention education may reinforce to teens that alcohol and drugs reduce good decision-making and impair brain development. As noted by one author, "Let youth be the only thing impairing their judgment."
- With the knowledge that mental health issues in teens are often undetected and unaddressed, maintain a vigilant watch for teens exhibiting any signs and symptoms and refer accordingly.
- Work to reduce the stigma of mental health issues.
- Assessing for drug, alcohol, and cigarette use and abuse and the extent of use are critical elements of the teen physical examination and in any history taking or health interaction with HCPs.

- Ingestion of drugs and alcohol during the earlier stages of adolescence increases the likelihood of dependence (those who start before they are 15 years of age are seven times more likely to become dependent). We recommend "just say later" instead of "just say no."
- It is important for adults to role model responsible drinking, to not condone illegal drug use or underage drinking, and to be vigilant for changes in teens' behaviors.
- In a health care system focused on crisis and intervention after the problem is significant, many support the need for prevention education, early screening, and timely intervention in managing emotional health issues in teens.

SUGGESTED READING

Carrion, V. G., Weems, C. F., & Reiss, A. L. (2007). Stress predicts brain changes in children: A pilot study on youth stress, PTSD, and the hippocampus. *Pediatrics, 119*(3), 509–516.

Chen, E., & Hanson, M. (2005). Perceptions of threat: Understanding pathways between stress and health in adolescents. *The Prevention Researcher, 12*(3), 10–12.

Corte, C., & Zucker, R. A. (2008). Self-concept disturbances: Cognitive vulnerability for early drinking & early drunkenness in adolescents at high risk for alcohol problems. *Addictive Behaviors, 33*, 1282–1290.

Davis, N. (2005). Depression in children and adolescence. *Journal of School Nursing, 21*(6), 311–317.

DiClemente, R. J., Santelli, J. S., & Crosby, R. A. (Eds.). (2009). *Adolescent health: Understanding and prevention risk behaviors.* San Francisco, CA: Jossey-Bass.

Falck, R. S., Nahhas, R. W., Li, L., & Carlson, R. G. (2012). Surveying teens in school to assess the prevalence of problem drug use. *Journal of Adolescent Health, 82*, 217–224.

Feinstein, E. C., Richter, L., & Foster, S. E. (2012). Addressing the critical health problems of adolescent substance use through health care, research, and public policy. *Journal of Adolescent Health, 50*, 431–436.

Feinstein, S. (2007). *Teaching the at-risk teenage brain.* Lanham, MD: Rowman & Littlefield.

Gardner, H. (2000). *Intelligence reframed: Multiple intelligences for the 21st century.* New York, NY: Basic Books.

Hamrin, V., & Magorino, M. (2010). Assessment of the adolescent for depression in the pediatric primary care setting. *Pediatric Nursing, 36*(2), 103–111.

Hayes, E., & Plowfield, L. (2007). Smoking too young: Students' decisions about tobacco use. *MCN: The American Journal of Maternal/Child Nursing, 32*(2), 112–116.

Herrman, J. (2005). The teen brain as a work in progress: Implications for pediatric nurses. *Pediatric Nursing, 31*, 144–148.

Howland, R. H. (2007). Antidepressants and suicide: Putting the risk in perspective. *Journal of Psychosocial Nursing, 45*(7), 15–19.

Johnson, S. B., Sudhinaraset, M., & Blum, R. W. (2010). Neuromaturation and adolescent risk taking: Why development is not determinism. *Journal of Adolescent Research, 25*(1), 4–23.

King, K. K., Strunk, C. M., & Sutter, M. T. (2011). Preliminary effectiveness of Surviving the Teens Suicide Prevention and Depression Awareness Program on adolescents' suicidality and self-efficacy in performing help-seeking behaviors. *Journal of School Health, 81*(9), 581–590.

LaRue, D., & Herrman, J. W. (2008). Adolescent stress through the eyes of high risk teens. *Pediatric Nursing, 34*, 375–380.

McNeely, C., & Blanchard, J. (2009). *The teen years explained: A guide to healthy adolescent development.* Baltimore, MD: Johns Hopkins Bloomburg School of Public Health.

Murphey, D., Barry, M., & Vaughn, B. (2013). *Adolescent health highlight: Mental health disorders.* Washington, DC: ChildTrends.

Puskar, K. R., Bernardo, L., Hatam, M., Geise, S., Bendik, K. J., & Grabiak, B. R. (2006). Self-cutting behaviors in adolescence. *Journal of Emergency Nursing, 32*(5), 444–446.

Serafini, T., Rye, B. J., & Drysdale, M. (Eds.). (2013). *Taking sides: Clashing views on adolescence.* New York, NY: McGraw-Hill.

Spear, L. P. (2000). Neurobehavioral changes in adolescence. *Current Directions in Psychological Science, 9*(4), 111–114.

Steinberg, L. (2008). *Adolescence.* New York, NY: McGraw-Hill.

SUGGESTED WEBSITES

Kids Health.Org
www.kidshealth.org/teen

Girl Scouts
www.girlscouts.org

AddHealth
www.cpc.unc.edu/projects/
addhealth

Child Trends
www.childtrends.org

The Bureau For At-Risk Youth
www.at-risk.com

National Clearinghouse on
Families and Youth
www.ncfy.acf.hhs.gov

Girls, Incorporated
www.girlsinc.org

Go Ask Alice
www.goaskalice.columbia.edu

Society for Adolescent
Medicine and Health
www.adolescenthealth.org

Healthy People
www.healthypeople.gov

Johns Hopkins School of
Public Health
www.jhsph.edu

Learn to Be Healthy
www.learntobehealthy.org/
teens

Office of Adolescent Health
www.hhs.gov/ash/oah

University of Minnesota Extension
http://www1.extension.umn
.edu/family/cyfc/our-services/

Teen Help.com
www.teenhelp.com

8

Spiritual Health

The concepts of religion and spirituality are not often part of health care interactions with youth or in addressing the health needs of teens. Ongoing research provides compelling evidence that teens who embrace spirituality and affiliate with religious practices may experience enhanced self-esteem, perceive feelings of higher levels of health, and exhibit positive health practices. Assessing and supporting spirituality and religious practices are key components of holistic care.

In this chapter, you will learn to:

1. Contrast the concepts of religion and spirituality
2. Discuss the stages of spiritual development
3. Analyze the impact of religiosity and spirituality on teen health
4. Identify key focused interventions based upon learned concepts

KEY DEFINITIONS

Adolescence is a time when teens begin to assess their own thoughts and those of others in their world that are related to spirituality and religion. Although not often addressed in health care, some believe that spirituality and religion are critical components of holistic practice and important to both physical and mental health. Some contend that one may be spiritual and not practice religion in the more formal sense, while others believe the two concepts are intertwined and difficult to separate. Adolescence is often when teens report having deep-seated spiritual beliefs but may pull away from formal religious practices and organizations. Teens tend to focus on the internal aspects of religion (beliefs, commitment) and less on the external signs, including going to church and affiliation with a specific religion. How adults understand teens' thoughts on spirituality and religion and ways to ensure health may be influenced by definitions of these concepts as described in Table 8.1.

Although these constructs are somewhat difficult to measure, recent research yields important data related to

TABLE 8.1 Comparing Spirituality and Religion

Spirituality	Religion
Connectedness with a higher being	May identify with a religious organization
Describes the meaning of life and includes personal dimensions on life and death	Characterized by formal practices, habits, and rituals
Includes thoughts, feelings, and beliefs	Characterized by a set of beliefs and practices shared by a group
Characterized by awe and reverence for that which is sacred	May have ethnic, regional, cultural, ancestral, or national commonalities
Describes the relationship among self, others, and a higher being	Manifested as outward practices of people related to beliefs and shared values

adolescents and their spirituality or involvement in religion. Table 8.2 shares data from the Monitoring the Future survey, a teen-focused study.

FAST FACTS in a NUTSHELL

- The numbers of youth attending religious services decreased from 2002 to 2006, reversing an increase in attendance in the previous decade.
- Little is known about the impact of gender on the spiritual development and religiosity in teens, indicating a potential area of ongoing study.

TABLE 8.2 Facts About Teens and Religion

- 84% of teens believed in God
- 55% of teens considered themselves spiritual but not religious
- 65% of teens prayed at least once per week
- 85% of teens considered themselves participants in a religious denomination (about 1/3 identified themselves as conservative Christian and 1/5 as Catholic)
- 42% of teens attended a religious function one time per week
- 52% of teens believed that their religious faith was important in shaping their daily life
- 39% of teens were in a youth group associated with a religious organization
- 48% of teens thought a religious organization was a good place to seek out help
- Younger teens (42%) were more likely to attend religious activities once per week than older teens (32%)
- African American teens (44%) were more likely to attend religious activities once per week than White teens (31%), and Hispanics reported slightly more participation in religious activities than Whites
- Wealthier teens (38%) were more likely to attend religious activities once a week than lower-income teens (28%)
- Rural teens tended to observe religious practices more than urban teens
- Teens in the South and Midwest attended more religious events than teens in other areas in the country
- College youth tended to be less affiliated with religious practices than teens of the same age who do not attend college

SPIRITUAL DEVELOPMENT

Our spirituality develops throughout our life span. It is generally agreed that spiritual development is shaped both by the beliefs, practices, and traditions of a religion and on the more existential thoughts and feelings associated with spirituality. Fowler identified six stages of spiritual development based on independent decision-making about how we think and feel, cognitive development, and a maturing sense of reason. The six stages are found in Table 8.3.

There are two stages in this model, with their characteristic behaviors, that pertain to teens:

Synthetic–Conventional Faith

- Teens are beginning to establish ideas about their own spiritual identity and tend to base these thoughts on the beliefs and actions of others.
- Teens are essentially striving to figure out who they are and are beginning to assess their own thoughts and beliefs.
- This phase is characterized by building on the thoughts, beliefs, practices, and traditions of others. Parents, adult role models, family, and peers are relied upon by teens to inform their thoughts on their spiritual identity.

TABLE 8.3 Stages of Spiritual Development

Stage	Ages	Stage Name
1	3–7 years	Intuitive–Protective Faith
2	Elementary school age	Mystical–Literal Faith
3	Adolescence	Synthetic–Conventional Faith
4	Late adolescence	Individualistic–Reflective Faith
5	Adulthood	Conjunctive Faith
6	Adulthood and beyond	Universalizing Faith

- Using the beliefs of others, teens build a personal belief system. Although youth may hold deep-seated beliefs about religion and spirituality, they have not yet critically examined or analyzed these values.

Individualistic–Reflective Faith

- As teens develop a more defined identity, they begin to question their own beliefs about religion and spirituality. Rather than simply doing and believing what parents and other adults tell them or role model for them in their lives, teens exert their independence and continue to refine their personal belief system.
- As the teen is more able to embrace abstract cognitive functions, the concept of spirituality takes on a more personal and conceptual process.
- Although some elements of spirituality are taken at face value, others are questioned as the teen continues to build a sense of reason.
- As teens question the values of others, discord about religious practices may result, especially with parents and other family members.
- Teens begin to value authenticity and consistency and question practices that seem to "not make sense" or contradict beliefs.
- Leadership by and esteem for adults at this stage are earned rather than appointed, so following religious traditions may be resisted during the teen years.
- The teen years may be characterized by searching for a faith that rings true to their personal needs and ideas about truth and spirituality.

In adulthood, during the stage of Conjunctive Faith, individuals begin to appreciate their own mortality, the need to accept things that cannot be changed, the inevitability of death, and the limitations of their personal abilities and identity. Fowler contended that only a rare few reach the final phase of Universalizing Faith, in which total selflessness and sacrifice transcend personal needs and aspirations.

IMPACT OF RELIGIOSITY AND SPIRITUALITY ON TEEN HEALTH

Spirituality and religiosity are important to adolescents as they navigate the teen years and make decisions about their health and behaviors. There is compelling evidence that spirituality is positively correlated with physical and mental health and that lower rates of physical morbidity and mortality are related to higher levels of self-reported religiosity. In adults, sources have noted better outcomes after surgery, a positive sense of purpose, improved coping skills, and higher ratings of overall well-being related to higher self-reports of spirituality. Religiosity and spirituality in teens have been noted to have a variety of positive outcomes, including:

- Assists in coping with chronic illness.
- May protect against depression.
- Enhances self-esteem in teens and assists teens in exploring their personal identity.
- Promotes positive self-care practices and self-rated health, which is correlated with future health.
- Fosters pro-social behaviors, leadership skills, altruism, and communication skills.
- Improves outcomes when being treated for mental health disorders.
- Promotes positive health behaviors.
- Provides positive adult role models.
- Protects against participation in risk behaviors. Religious attendance has been found to be related to decreased cigarette smoking, use of alcohol, use of marijuana, engagement in premarital intercourse, or engagement in delinquent behavior. These protective mechanisms may be especially powerful in minority and low-income teens.
- Promotes positive peer relations and role modeling.

- Prayer and meditation were associated with increased blood flow to the brain, potentially allowing for increased mental focus and reasoning skills.
- Religion and spirituality may be related to more positive family relations, which were associated with positive school performance.
- Research demonstrates that active participation in the practices of a religious organization and working with the people in a religious organization were more protective than the private practice of prayer and spirituality.

In summary, involvement in religion is most often associated with positive health behaviors and plays an important role in guiding health decision-making. For example, participation in religious organizations has been found to protect inner-city youth from the harmful effects of community violence and poverty. Some resources contend that, rather than religiosity being the positive factor, it is actually positive relationships with parents, long-lasting attachments with people in their world, the presence of positive adult role models, and pro-social peer relationships that foster these positive impacts. Organized religion may have negative impacts on the self-esteem of youth if their lifestyles or gender orientation may oppose religious tenets. Teens who are gay, lesbian, bisexual, or questioning, already going through difficult self-searching, may receive reduced support or rejection from religious organizations. Health care providers need to assess teens' needs for support and information as they explore their sexual orientation.

FOCUSED INTERVENTIONS

- Include religion and spirituality as part of our uniform assessment of youth.
- Few formal tools exist for use with teens to assess spirituality and religiosity. Two adult scales, the Spiritual Involvement and Beliefs Scale (SIBS) and the Spiritual Well-Being Scale (SWBS), may be useful in

preliminary assessments of these concepts with teens (see Rubin, Dodd, Desai, Pollock, & Graham-Pole, 2009).

- Allow teens to discuss their thoughts on spirituality and religion and how choices in those areas may impact their health.
- Assess for personal and family decision-making, as it may impact personal lifestyle issues or life decisions, including sexual orientation, gender orientation, sexual behavior, contraception, abortion, and others.
- Support teens as they develop their personal definition of social justice and their devotion to good for self and others. Service projects and doing for others are correlated with increased feelings of self-worth and decreased engagement in risk behaviors.
- Encourage exposure to a variety of experiences of spirituality, including journaling, artwork, literature, poetry, music, painting, and drama.
- Reassure parents that teens' exploration of new and different religions, changes in religious practices, and potentially controversial, expressed beliefs are a natural part of teen development and are part of the questioning and searching for personal identity inherent to the teen years. Some parents may see this as rebellion or their teen being difficult. Parents may benefit from information and support during this time.

SUGGESTED READING

ChildTrends. (2006). *Monitoring the future survey data 1976–2006.* Retrieved from http://www.Childtrends.org

Fowler, J. (1995). *Stages of faith: The psychology of human development.* New York, NY: Harper.

McNeely, C., & Blanchard, J. (2009). *The teen years explained: A guide to healthy adolescent development.* Baltimore, MD: Johns Hopkins Bloomburg School of Public Health.

Powell-Young, U. (2012). Household income and spiritual well-being but not body mass index as determinants of poor self-rated health among African-American adolescents. *Research in Nursing and Health, 35,* 219–230.

Rubin, D., Dodd, M., Desai, N., Pollock, B., & Graham-Pole, J. (2009). Spirituality in well and ill adolescents and their parents: The use of two assessment scales. *Pediatric Nursing, 35*(10), 37–42.

Steinberg, L. (2008). *Adolescence.* New York, NY: McGraw-Hill.

SUGGESTED WEBSITES

Advocates for Youth
www.advocatesforyouth.org

AddHealth
www.cpc.unc.edu/projects/
addhealth

Go Ask Alice
www.goaskalice.columbia
.edu

National Study of Youth and
Religion
www.youthandreligion.org

Healthy People
www.healthypeople.gov

Johns Hopkins School of
Public Health
www.jhsph.edu

9

Sexual Health and Risks

Gender influences much of how we exist in society. Gender transcends sexuality and impacts our actions and behaviors. Sexuality and sexual activity are a wonderful part of being human, yet adults are sometimes uncomfortable about teen sexuality, educating teens about sexual activity, and assisting teens to be healthy sexually. Nonetheless, it is a critical element of health, and unhealthy or unsafe sexual practices may take a toll on individuals and society.

In this chapter, you will learn to:

1. Discuss gender and the positive nature of teen sexual health
2. Address teen sexual activity and contraception
3. Analyze selected consequences of unsafe or unprotected sexual practices
4. Identify key focused interventions based upon learned concepts

GENDER

Gender is one of the traits that defines personal identity, guides decisions and behavior, and impacts adolescent development. It is believed that hormones influence brain maturation and that estrogen and testosterone stimulate the brain's emotional center, the limbic system, leading to potential mood changes and sensation seeking. It is important to note that individuals are impacted by many influences in addition to gender. Environment, learning and experience, genetics, and nutrition, in addition to brain development, influence behavior in individuals. The potential differences in the male and female brain and their effects on behavior are being explored. Table 9.1 describes selected differences manifested by the two genders.

TABLE 9.1 Gender Differences

Girls	Boys
Estrogen fosters communication, nurturing, and social bonds; protects from stress	Testosterone fosters aggression, achievement, and sexual activity; suppresses pruning
Priorities: attractiveness, approval, and social connection (tend and befriend)	Priorities: authority, accomplishment, and isolation (fight or flight)
Girls are thought to see relationships and protection as paramount related to their reproductive capacity	Males appear to be more focused on concerns outside the family and are more adventurous
Like to avoid conflict	Like to confront conflict
Speak an average of 250 words/minute	Speak an average of 125 words/minute
Activities may be more influenced by potential consequences	Activities may be more impulsive without consideration of consequences
Tend to be empathizing—focus on relationships	Tend to be systemizing—focus on detail and productiveness
Girls' brains mature around 1½ years prior to boys'	Boys' brains mature later than girls' brains, especially in proliferation and pruning
Female brains have larger basal ganglia, larger corpus callosum, and increased blood flow over males	These differences may explain selected differences in male and female skills and talents

Development of sexual and gender identity, as part of the larger task of identity formation, is a confusing time and is influenced by genetics, family, friends, and context. Table 9.2 provides important definitions about gender and sexual orientation.

TABLE 9.2 Gender and Sexual Orientation Definitions

Gender identity	A person's internal, deeply felt sense of being male, female, other, or in between. Everyone has a gender identity.
Gender role behavior	The prevailing societal expectations of how individuals behave based on gender. This is highly impacted by norms, values, and practices of a group.
Sexual orientation	A person's emotional and sexual attraction to other people based on the gender of the person. A person may identify his or her sexual orientation as heterosexual, lesbian, gay, bisexual, or queer.
Gender expression	Characteristics that are perceived as masculine and feminine, such as appearance, speech, dress, or social interactions.
Transgender	People whose gender identity, characteristics, or expression do not conform to the identity or characteristics of their biological sex.
LBGTQ	An umbrella term for lesbian, bisexual, gay, transgender, and questioning. Questioning refers to those who are not yet certain of their sexual or gender identity.
Transsexual	A person who identifies with behaviors different from his or her biological sex. May include how one dresses, surgical revision, or other changes.
Homosexual or gay	A person whose sexual and emotional feelings are mostly for people of the same sex.
Heterosexual or straight	A person whose sexual and emotional feelings are mostly for people of the opposite sex.
Bisexual	A person whose sexual and emotional feelings are for males and females.
Lesbian	A homosexual woman.
Queer	A term that used to be negative; now a positive term used for LGBTQ or those who do not conform to traditional norms of gender or sexuality.

Gender places certain stressors on teens as they develop physically and sexually. Supportive adults need to be sensitive of teens as they develop and may question their gender identity and sexual orientation. Teens may engage in same-sex play and think about their sexual preferences. About 8% of boys and 6% of girls report being attracted to someone of the same sex during their teen years; by age 19 about 5% of males and 14% of females report having at least one same-sex encounter with a sex partner. It is believed that girls are more accustomed to being intimate with other girls on an emotional level whereas boys tend to be wary of such emotions or closeness. Researchers contend that this may be the origin of "homophobia" among boys who feel less comfortable with the expression of sexuality toward same-sex partners. Adolescent preferences may or may not persist in adulthood; about 3% to 5% of adults report being gay or lesbian.

TEEN SEXUALITY AND SEXUAL HEALTH

Development of a sexual self is a normal part of adolescent maturation. Sexual development includes such components as self-esteem, body image, gender identity, and gender role behavior. Sexual socialization is a product of how children are exposed to and educated about sexuality. Part of physical development is measured through the acquisition of secondary sexual characteristics and gaining the ability to reproduce. Sexuality, or an individual's ability to function sexually and the associated emotions, is a key part of being human and is critical across the life span. Several influences may impact development and ongoing perceptions of sexuality, including personal expectations, family, culture, and religion. Although often considered a political "hot potato," teen sexuality is an important part of learning to relate to others, developing intimacy with another person, demonstrating intimacy through sexual means, and expressing love and devotion to another human being. Because almost 80% of teens have had sex upon leaving high school, perhaps we should reframe teen sexual activity as a normative experience that is a choice for some, but not all, teens.

Rather than viewing sexuality as something to be accrued when one turns 18 or the age of majority, the characteristics of sexuality and sexual milestones begin at birth and continue throughout the life span. By being aware of these stages, parents and other key role models may ensure that teens are fully informed about their sexual development and also about the values, rules, and expectations of the family, their religious or spiritual affiliations, and their culture (Table 9.3).

TABLE 9.3 Stages of the Development of Sexuality

Infants and toddlers	Beginning knowledge of body parts and personal boundaries Exploration of pleasure and tactile stimulation Linking of loving and emotions with physical touch
Preschool and school age	Learning about body part functions and ways to enhance or cause pleasure (masturbation) Learning about appropriate behavior in certain settings and with certain individuals Ongoing development of personal boundaries Beginning feelings of sexual attraction and "puppy love" or crushes as experiments for future relationships Beginning of sexual and romantic fantasies Understanding and feeling comfortable with the body May have many questions about sexuality and sexual activity
Early teen years	Hormones of puberty stimulate feelings of sexuality and perceiving one's self as a sexual being Changes in hormone levels change appearance, impacting self-concept and self-esteem Beginning exploration of sexual media Increased curiosity about sex and sexual activity Understanding and feeling comfortable with one's changing and developing body Accepting one's own feelings of sexual arousal and associated stimuli (continued masturbation and self-stimulation)

(continued)

TABLE 9.3 Stages of the Development of Sexuality (*continued*)

Mid-teen years	Ongoing adaptation to changing body and sexual feelings
	Ongoing exploration of sexual media (books, Internet, movies, social media)
	Teens may experience increased sex drive, more thoughts about sex, and more interest in romance
	Cognitive development allows teens to reflect on sexual thoughts and behaviors
	Making choices about sexual activity
	Early understanding of and potential for practicing safe sex
Late adolescence and early adulthood	Physical development is usually complete
	Intimacy and relationships may be associated with sexual activity
	Understanding and practicing safe sexual activity
	Continued maturation of personal and partners' sexual desires and preferred practices
	Ongoing development of emotional and romantic elements associated with sexual activity
	Increased emphasis on pleasuring of others before self
Adulthood and elder adulthood	Continued maturation of personal and partners' sexual desires and preferred practices
	Ongoing development of emotional and romantic elements associated with sexual activity
	Increased emphasis on pleasuring of others before self
	Acceptance of changing sexual practices associated with physical ability and maturation

These stages may differ based on culture, ages of maturation, and cognitive and emotional development. Adults often have a difficult time communicating with teens about sex and may need to research some questions they don't know how to answer. It is better to say you don't know something rather than demeaning the teen's question or conjuring up an incorrect answer. Teens with developmental disabilities, and their families, often have to deal with a body that is physically mature plus an even greater chasm than most teens between this physical maturity and cognitive abilities to control impulses and understand their changing bodies.

Sexual Activity

Sexual experience is a natural part of growing up. When sexual activity begins is based on individual desires, personal values, opportunity, the readiness for intimacy, parent–child communication, peer pressure, hormonal urges, curiosity, and religious values. Additional factors believed to initiate or increase teen sexual activity include believing friends are sexually active, the media, decreased parental supervision/monitoring, sexually active siblings, siblings having babies, living in a single-parent family, and early-maturing individuals. Some believe that males tend to begin their sexual lives seeing sexual activity as a recreational, and emotional, activity. Because boys tend to have masturbated and may have experienced orgasms, or had nocturnal emissions, prior to sexual activity, they are familiar with sexual pleasure and may see sexual activity as different from intimacy. Girls are not as likely to have masturbated, so sexual activity may be their first experience with orgasms. They may consider love and romance associated with sexual activity and may be more cognizant of the consequences of sexual activity, including pregnancy. These facts may impact how teens approach their early sexual experiences.

The rate of teens engaging in sexual activity has actually reduced since the 1980s and 1990s. Although the rate is lower, significant areas of concern continue to play into the controversies over teen sexual activity, as cited in Table 9.4.

Sexuality Education

If you ask most adults where they learned about sex, they often say friends, parents, siblings, books, and other experiences. This has changed dramatically in current times, where parents and family, the media, the Internet, and school play large roles in sexuality education. Teens report that they are more likely to get information about contraceptives from the Internet than

U.S. rates of teen sexual activity:

- 47.4% of all high school students had sexual intercourse.
- 20% of teens leaving high school do not participate in sexual activity (80% do).
- 34% of teens had sex in the past 3 months prior (decreased 10% since 1991).
- 20% of girls and 30% of boys 15 years or less are sexually active.
- 15.3% of teens had four or more sex partners.
- 20% to 25% of teens used drugs or alcohol with their last sexual activity.
- 78% of teens use contraception at the first sexual encounter.
- 63% of teens used a condom at last intercourse (up from 46% in 1991).
- 54% of female teens are sexually active, with 60% using highly effective contraception and 18% not using any contraception.
- 43% of never-married teen girls and 42% of never-married teen boys reported experiencing sexual intercourse.
- 70% to 90% of teen sexual activity is voluntary, but 25% may be considered unwanted.
- Without use of contraception for 1 year, sexually active young women have a 90% chance of sustaining a pregnancy.

asking their parents or health care providers. Although 75% of prime-time television shows include sexual innuendos or content, only about 10% mention safe sex practices. In many ways the media has replaced parents for information, and studies tell us that teens watching sexually explicit material are twice as likely to engage in sexual activity. Although advertisements on television depict erectile dysfunction and other personal products, TV stations have yet to allow advertising for condoms, emergency contraception, or birth control.

TABLE 9.4 Areas of Concern About Teen Sexual Activity

- The ability of teens to cognitively understand and control sexual behaviors and practice safe sexual behaviors
- Teens' abilities to comprehend the responsibilities and consequences associated with unprotected sexual activity
- The impact of drugs and alcohol on sexual decision-making and activity and the potential for date-rape drugs to lead to unwanted sexual activity
- The declining age of sexual activity, especially among girls and early-maturing teens
- The increased disclosure of child sexual exploitation or abuse and the potential for increased premature and unsafe sexual behaviors among victims
- What exactly is included in sexual activity—vaginal intercourse, anal sex, oral sex, use of sexually stimulating devices, etc.
- The relationship of emotions, love, and devotion to sexual activity
- The lessening emphasis on the personal nature of sexual activity
- Sexual activity between younger girls and older male partners
- The potential for coercion, involuntary sexual activity, and reproductive/contraceptive sabotage using sexual activity in power struggles within relationships
- Racial and ethnic disparities of sexual activity, use of contraception or protection, and reports of unintended pregnancies or sexually transmitted infections (STIs)
- The relationship of other high-risk behaviors with risky sexual behaviors (including school truancy or failure, use of drugs and alcohol, sexual and child abuse, involvement in juvenile justice, domestic violence, etc.)
- The potential that mental health issues, poor coping skills, or increased life stresses may lead to premature or unsafe sexual experiences
- Lack of parental monitoring, parent–child relationships, or communication about sexual activity and safe sexual behavior
- Changes in family structure, family values, or religiosity that may influence sexual decision-making and promote responsible sexual behaviors
- Many teens practice serial monogamy wherein they have sexual relationships with one partner at a time but may have several intense relationships in the teen years
- 30% of teens report being involved in a "friends with benefits" relationship where sexual activity may occur in nonromantic relationships

Sexuality education is paramount in order to assist teens to navigate their sexuality safely. Unfortunately, sexuality education in the United States often comes too late in the high school years and the content is riddled with controversy. Despite the fact that there is overwhelming public support to teach both abstinence and contraception to high school children, many school districts do not allow the discussion of condoms, contraception, and sexual activity. Health care providers may serve as youth advocates in their community, in addition to serving as information sources, to ensure optimal sexuality education.

There are significant misconceptions about sex. Research about teens' knowledge of sexuality revealed some surprising findings, as found in Table 9.5, and reinforces the need for medically accurate, developmentally appropriate, and culturally sensitive sexuality education.

When asking teens about what they want in teen pregnancy–prevention programs, they appear to agree that they want honest, factual information about the structure and function of the human body, the means to be safe when having sex, ways to deal with peer pressure, and about sexually transmitted infections (STIs) and pregnancy. Teens don't want to be told to have or not to have sex; they want to learn

TABLE 9.5 Selected Teen Misconceptions About Sex

Question	Answer	% Correct
1 Teens cannot get pregnant the first time they have sex	False	73%
2 In an emergency it is okay to use someone else's birth control pills	False	50%
3 Urinating after sex may prevent pregnancy	False	39%
4 Sperm can live for a few days in the woman's body	True	41%
5 Douching is a method of birth control	False	30%
6 Letting sperm drip out after sex prevents pregnancy	False	26%
7 A female can get pregnant through oral sex	False	44%

Source: Carrera, Kaye, Philliber, and West (2000).

about good decision-making, how to negotiate sexual experiences, and the value of and personal efforts needed in relationships. Teens and adults agree that boys and girls need to learn about safe sexual behaviors. Sometimes it appears that prevention efforts are focused on girls. Just as it takes two to conceive a baby, it should take all partners to prevent conception and be safe during sexual activity. Heterosexual and homosexual teens need to learn about protection and responsible sexual behavior. Although the focus of sexuality classes for teens who are LGBTQ may be on disease prevention, the high rate of teen pregnancy among lesbian and questioning girls warrants additional pregnancy prevention efforts.

Prevention strategies that support responsible sexual behaviors promote delaying sexual initiation, decreasing frequency of sexual experiences, relationship skills, decreasing the number of sexual partners, increasing condom use, and increasing use of other contraceptives. Many curricula and programs exist and current emphasis is placed on those that are evidence-based, medically accurate, culturally acceptable, developmentally appropriate, and teen friendly. Kirby, Rollieri, and Wilson (2007) identified 17 characteristics of effective teen pregnancy prevention programs that may be helpful to those developing, implementing, or evaluating prevention programs in their community.

Although some adults fear that sexuality education, teen pregnancy prevention initiatives, and providing access to birth control may increase levels of teen sexual activity, this is not the case. Research demonstrates that such programs increase safe sexual practices in sexually active youth but do not increase the percentage of teens engaging in sexual activity. In fact, some contend that access to information and reproductive health services decreases teen sexual activity and delays sexual initiation. Programs to prevent teen pregnancy, teach about relationships, and promote responsible sexual behavior may take place in a variety of settings. Different venues for and types of teen pregnancy prevention initiatives are listed in Table 9.6.

Although highly values based, some contend that sexuality between consenting adults has few boundaries. Although this issue becomes more complex with teens, it is when sexual

TABLE 9.6 Venues for and Types of Teen Pregnancy Prevention Strategies

Nurse home-visiting programs	Community clinics
Family planning services	Advance provision of emergency contraception
School-based health center provision of contraception	Teen mother/grandmother/teen father/grandfather and sibling programs
Teen parent testimonials	
School condom availability programs	Peer counseling programs
Youth development programs	Mentoring programs
Life option/goal setting/career programs	Service learning programs
Smart phone or texting programs	Community-wide programs
Video- or computer-based programs	School-based sex education
Media awareness campaigns	Decision-making initiatives
Programs to prevent or delay subsequent pregnancy in young parents	Educating about the consequences of teen parenting

activity becomes coercive, uncomfortable, or involuntary that the sexual act may become abusive. It is reported that for 10% to 30% of girls, their first sexual experience is involuntary, whether through coercion, date rape, abuse, under the influence of drugs or alcohol, or incest. Others discuss the fact that, for some teens, sex is voluntary but not wanted. About 25% of sexually active young women wish they had waited longer, delayed sexual activity, or state that their first sexual experience was unpleasant or under duress. Communication is critical in order to ensure partners are gratified by the sexual experience, that the acts are part of each individual's free will, and that there is no remorse following the actions.

Contraception, Protection, and Abortion

Teens who are sexually active need contraceptives that are easily accessible, require low effort for use, and that they are motivated to use in order to prevent unintended pregnancy and the communicability of STIs. Descriptions and benefits of types of birth control for teens are noted in Table 9.7.

TABLE 9.7 Contraception Methods Used by Teens

Male condoms	• Accessible without a prescription • Relatively easy to use—need to be applied and removed correctly, checked for intactness, and expiration date • Inexpensive • Must stay in place during entire sexual act • Must be part of pre-planning and available during sexual encounter • Some partners do not accept their use or oppose use due to changes in perceptions of pleasure • Protect against pregnancy and STIs
Female condoms	• Less socially accepted and may be difficult for teens to use; may make noise during sexual activity • Enable female to control protection • Need to be inserted and removed correctly, checked for intactness, and expiration date • More expensive than male condoms • Protect against pregnancy and STIs
Hormone methods	• Pills, patches, injections, vaginal ring, and implanted methods • Change the hormonal environment, inhibit ovulation, and make the uterine wall less suitable for implantation • Require vigilant reapplication, taking pills, injections, or insertion based on timed schedules • Is implemented away from the sexual act and allows for spontaneity and separation of the contraception from sexual activity (noncoital method) • May produce side effects • More costly and require prescription • Do not protect against STIs • Increased emphasis is currently placed on long-acting reversible contraceptives (LARCs) with teens, including implanted and injected hormones or intrauterine devices to prevent teen pregnancy • Emergency contraceptives (Plan B) are hormonal formulations that prevent an unplanned pregnancy after unprotected sexual activity. Must be used within 72 hours of unprotected sexual activity and is available over-the-counter for some teens. Many health care providers recommend that, due to the potential for disturbing side effects and the need to adhere to the regimen, teens may benefit from consultation with an adult or health care provider when using Plan B

(continued)

TABLE 9.7 Contraception Methods Used by Teens (continued)	
Barrier methods	• Diaphragm, cervical cap, and intrauterine devices create a mechanical or chemical barrier to fertilization • Some barrier methods need to be applied prior to sexual activity and left in place for a certain duration after intercourse • Dental dams or impermeable barriers may prevent exposure to STIs during oral sex • Require comfort with body, prescription, and some level of personal effort to ensure protection • Do not protect against STIs
Natural methods	• Withdrawal, calculating safe times for pregnancy without fertilization, breastfeeding, and the rhythm method are not effective in preventing pregnancy or STI transmission • These methods are even less effective with teens because of their inability to pre-plan, adhere to method stipulations, or adhere to time and behavior restrictions

Abortion is legal in all 50 states in the United States. Some state regulations related to abortion procedures are changing such that state laws about parental consent, waiting periods, father consent, and the age of consent for a therapeutic abortion or pregnancy termination differ. Health care providers should be aware of the restrictions within their state of practice.

TEEN PREGNANCY, STIs, AND HIV

About 750,000 pregnancies occur among teens each year. These pregnancies are associated with racial, ethnic, geographic, and economic disparities. About half of these pregnancies lead to births, about one third are terminated, and the balance represent miscarriages, with only about 1% to 2% of the children of teen pregnancies adopted. The teen pregnancy rate in the United States is about nine times higher than other developed, industrialized countries in the world.

The teen pregnancy rate has decreased 40% from 1990 to 2008 and the teen birth rate has declined 49% since 1991

- Teen pregnancy rate is 70 per 1,000; the teen birth rate is 42 per 1,000
- 10% of the births in the United States are to teens
- 10% of teens experience a pregnancy; 19% of sexually active teens become pregnant
- 90% of teen pregnancies are unintended
- 10% of teen mothers marry the father of their child
- 1.6 million teen pregnancies are averted each year due to contraceptive use
- 19 million new STIs are diagnosed each year; half of these are in youth 15 to 24 years of age, even though they make up only 25% of the sexually active individuals
- 25% of sexually active teens have been diagnosed with STIs
- 25% of those diagnosed with HIV are less than 25 years of age

and 25% from 2007 to 2011, reflecting rates that are at historic lows. These declines in rates are attributed to both a decrease in teen participation in sexual activity (20% of the decline) and to more effective use of contraception (80% of the decline). National research substantiated that most teen pregnancies are unintended, yet almost one half of all teens were not using birth control and one third thought they could not get pregnant at the time of sexual activity.

The inherent risk of contracting an STI or HIV from single or multiple sexual partners is evident. Sexually transmitted infections may lead to infected babies, pelvic inflammatory disease, and reproductive dysfunction. Most STIs can be treated with antimicrobials. Viral infections, like herpes and human papilloma virus (HPV), are not curable but may be treated symptomatically. The HPV vaccine is now recommended for young women prior to sexual activity and experts recommend young men also receive the vaccine

One of the greatest risks associated with sexual activity is the actual exposure to others and their partners. It is conjectured that sexual exposures are exponential such that an individual with 5 sexual partners is exposed to 31 other individuals, and even more shocking, a teen with 12 partners is exposed to 4,095 partners!

in order to prevent HPV; the vaccine can also prevent some forms of cervical cancer. HIV, though considered at this time a treatable disease, is not curable and demands a life-long course of treatment with many sequelae.

TEEN PARENTING

Although teen sexual activity and pregnancy may include areas of controversy, health care providers are often called upon to provide care to teen parents. Not only are the teen parents our patients, but their children are also important new patients who need our care! Marriage between teen partners who find they are pregnant used to be the norm, with 80% marrying during pregnancy. As economic and social issues have changed, marriage is no longer the norm, with less than 10% marrying. Many teen parents are highly caring and work hard to be good parents. These young parents may need extra support, information, and resources in order to optimize their abilities. In fact, support from parents or others is the single most common mitigating factor and predicts the success of the young parents. In converse, sources of help that stifle the young parents in their development of parenting skills and independence may have a negative impact. The perfect balance of help and independence is difficult to attain but so important to help young parents. Table 9.8 cites some of the issues confronted by young parents. One unresolved perspective is whether poverty leads to teen pregnancy or whether teen pregnancy predisposes an individual to living in poverty. Perhaps it suffices to say that they are strongly correlated and difficult to address when they occur together.

TABLE 9.8 Potential Issues Confronted by Young Parents

- Although thought by some to be overstated, early childrearing has some significant consequences:
  - For the mother: Only 60% graduate high school and 30% graduate college before they turn 30 years of age. This may set the woman up for a life of inability to self-sustain economically, dependence on a male, family, or federal subsidies, and poverty; subsequent pregnancy may exacerbate these issues with 20%–30% of all teen births being second or higher-order births; teen mothers are at increased risk of depression and intimate partner violence
  - For the father: Lower self-esteem, school performance, and school attendance; may have increased risk for substance use and patterns of delinquency; financial stressors associated with child support and family financial demands
  - For the child: The health of the babies of young mothers is dependent upon the mother's use of prenatal care (30% of teen mothers have inadequate prenatal care) and behaviors during pregnancy (drugs, alcohol, tobacco, nutrition, and health behaviors). Lack of screening and education or involvement in risk behaviors may lead to low birth weight, premature, or at-risk neonates. Children of teen parents have increased risk for hospitalization, school issues, and becoming teen parents themselves
  - For the community: May suffer if resources for young parents drain fiscal funds, less employed parents reduce the tax base, and teen pregnancy and parenting become a social norm
- Teens asked to evaluate the costs and rewards of teen parenting report that teen parenting would be "hard" and limit their social life, school activities, financial abilities, sleep, and daily activities
- Some teens consider the positive aspects of a teen birth, including getting more attention, having someone to love, the prospects of keeping one's partner, and the chance to make a positive contribution to the world. Research further informs us that young women living in disadvantage may not have hope of college or a career. For these young people a baby may affirm their future goals, give them purpose to work toward those goals, provide a positive and loving aspect as part of their lives, and ensure mothers turn around previous negative behaviors

FOCUSED INTERVENTIONS

- Health care providers are in a unique position to be knowledgeable and trusted by teens with regard to sexuality issues. We should respond with candidness and promote healthy behaviors without judgment or bias.

- One successful strategy to involve young parents and to encourage teens to make good decisions about sexual behavior is to have the young parents share their experiences as part of youth health classes, teen pregnancy prevention strategies, and encounters dealing with safe sexual behavior. Providing important messages about making goals for the future, planning ways to meet these goals, and delaying childrearing are critical.

- Use "invented dialogues" to provide teens with a ready response to those who make them uncomfortable about sex or pressure them to do things they do not want to do. Having a ready response to the requests of others, for example, "I have decided to wait until I get out of high school to have sex," allows teens to be prepared for these confrontations.

- When working with youth who are transgender or transsexual, ask them the names and pronouns they prefer. Provide the appropriate levels of privacy and support, including their choice of rest rooms and other accommodations to ensure their comfort.

- Sex education is a complex issue and the data suggest that a combination of promoting abstinence and information on contraception will have the best outcomes for the greatest number of teens. Make sure parents have the comfort level, knowledge, skills, and tools to provide sex and sexuality education to their teens.

- Methods to promote responsible sexual behavior and prevent teen pregnancy should be male and female focused. Strategies should reinforce the role of genders and need for all members of the sexual experience to act responsibly.

- Teen sex is most likely to happen at home when parents are working or not home. Supervision of free time, parental monitoring, and honest communication about expectations and safe sexual behavior are pivotal in preventing unsafe sexual practices.
- Contraceptive methods and recommendations change frequently and require that health care providers stay current on new methods of birth control and agents designed to promote safe sex.
- Adults who support access to birth control at age-appropriate times should consider issues of transportation, cost, service-related barriers, teens' development levels and abilities; consent issues; and maintain privacy and confidentiality in assisting teens to engage in responsible sexual behavior.
- Support teen parents during a very stressful time in their lives. Ensure that they have the knowledge and skills to parent, in addition to the resources, and be available to provide support and information as needed.
- In all interactions about sex and sexuality with teens, reinforce the beautiful and positive parts of sexuality, the associated responsibilities, and the sexuality in everyone, rather than the consequences, restrictions, or negative parts of the sexual experience!

SUGGESTED READING

Aquilini, M. L., & Bragadottir, H. (2000). Adolescent pregnancy: Teen perspectives on prevention. *MCN: The American Journal of Maternal/Child Nursing, 25*, 192–197.

Blakemore, S. J., & Choudhury, S. (2006). Development of the adolescent brain: Implications for executive function and social cognition. *Journal of Child Psychology and Psychiatry, 47*(3/4), 296–312.

Carrera, M., Kaye, J. W., Philliber, S., & West, E. (2000). Knowledge about reproduction, contraception, and sexually transmitted infections among young adolescents in American cities. *Social Policy, 30*, 41–50.

Center for Drug and Alcohol Studies, University of Delaware (CDAS). (2010). *Delaware high school survey: Risk behaviors and academic performance report.* Newark, DE: Author.

Centers for Disease Control and Prevention (CDC). (2012). Pre-pregnancy contraceptive use among teens with unintended pregnancy resulting in live births—PRAMS, 2004–2008. *Morbidity and Mortality Weekly Report, 61*(2), 25–29.

Centers for Disease Control and Prevention (CDC). (2012). Sexual experience and contraceptive use among female teens, US, 1995, 2002, & 2006–2012. *Morbidity and Mortality Weekly Report, 61*(17), 297–301.

Christopherson, T. M., & Conner, B. T. (2012). Mediation of late adolescent health-risk behaviors and gender influence. *Public Health Nursing, 29,* 510–524.

DeBellis, M. D., Keshavan, M. S., Beers, S. R., Hall, J., Frustaci, K., Masalehdan, A., . . . Boring, A. M. (2001). Sex differences in brain maturation during childhood and adolescence. *Cerebral Cortex, 11,* 552–557.

DiClemente, R. J., Santelli, J. S., & Crosby, R. A. (Eds.). (2009). *Adolescent health: Understanding and prevention risk behaviors.* San Francisco, CA: Jossey-Bass.

Doswell, W. M., & Braxter, B. (2002). Risk-taking behaviors in early adolescent minority women: Implications for research and practice. *Journal of Obstetric, Gynecologic, and Neonatal Nursing, 31,* 454–461.

Herrman, J. W. (2006). Position statement on the role of the pediatric nurse working with sexually active teens, pregnant adolescents, and young parents. *Journal of Pediatric Nursing, 21*(3), 250–252.

Herrman, J. W. (2006). The voices of teen mothers: The experience of repeat pregnancy. *MCN: The American Journal of Maternal/Child Nursing, 31*(4), 243–249.

Herrman, J. W. (2007). Repeat pregnancy in adolescence: Intentions and decision making. *MCN: The American Journal of Maternal/Child Nursing, 32*(2), 89–94.

Herrman, J. W. (2008). Adolescent perceptions of teen births: A focus group study. *Journal of Obstetrical, Gynecological, and Neonatal Nursing, 37*(1), 42–50.

Herrman, J. W. (2010). Assessing the teen parent family: The role for nurses. *Nursing for Women's Health, 14*(3), 212–221.

Herrman, J. W., & Waterhouse, J. K. (2011). What do adolescents think of teen parenting? *Western Journal of Nursing Research, 33*(4), 577–592.

Herrman, J. W., Solano, P., Stotz, L., & McDuffie, M. J. (2013). Comprehensive sexuality education: A historical and comparative analysis of public opinion. *American Journal of Sexuality Education, 8,* 140–159.

Kirby, D. B. (2007). *Emerging answers 2007: Research findings for programs to reduce teen pregnancy and sexually transmitted diseases.* Washington, DC: National Campaign to Prevent Teen and Unplanned Pregnancy.

Kirby, D. B., Rollieri, L., & Wilson, M. (2007). *Tools to assess the characteristics of effective sexuality and STD/HIV educational programs.* Washington, DC: Healthy Teen Network.

Martinez, G., Copen, C. E., & Abma J. C. (2011). Teenagers in the United States: Sexual activity, contraceptive use, and childbearing, 2006–2010 National Survey of Family Growth. National Center for Health Statistics. *Vital Health Statistics, 23*(31), 31–35.

McNeely, C., & Blanchard, J. (2009). *The teen years explained: A guide to healthy adolescent development.* Baltimore, MD: Johns Hopkins Bloomburg School of Public Health.

National Campaign to Prevent Teen and Unplanned Pregnancy. (2012). *Policy brief: Key points about teen pregnancy prevention.* Washington, DC: Author.

Steinberg, L. (2008). *Adolescence.* New York, NY: McGraw-Hill.

Terzian, M., & Moore, K. A. (2012). *Examining state-level patterns in teen childbearing: 1991–2009.* Washington, DC: ChildTrends.

SUGGESTED WEBSITES

Kids Health.Org
www.kidshealth.org/teen

Advocates for Youth
www.advocatesforyouth.org

The National Campaign to
Prevent Teen and
Unplanned Pregnancy
www.nationalcampaign.org

The Bureau For At-Risk Youth
www.at-risk.com

Centers for Disease Control
and Prevention
www.cdc.gov/healthyyouth

Children's Hospital of Boston
www.childrenshospital.org

Healthy People
www.healthypeople.gov

The Urban Institute
www.urban.org

CityMatch
www.citymatch.org

Healthy Teen Network
www.healthyteennetwork
.org

Guttmacher Foundation
www.guttmacher.org

SEICUS
www.seicus.org
Kaiser Foundation
www.kff.org
Childtrends
www.childtrends.org
The Search Institute
www.search-institute.org
National Clearinghouse on
Families and Youth
www.ncfy.acf.hhs.gov
Girls, Incorporated
www.girlsinc.org
Go Ask Alice
www.goaskalice.columbia.edu

Society for Adolescent
Medicine and Health
www.adolescenthealth.org
Johns Hopkins School of
Public Health
www.jhsph.edu
The Dibble Fund
www.dibblefund.org
Office of Adolescent Health
www.hhs.gov/ash/oah
YouthResource.com
www.youthresource.com
Teen Help.com
www.teenhelp.com

10

Relational Health and Risks

How teens relate socially has great bearing on their ability to be safe, happy, and effective in the world. Teens begin their social development within the constellation of their family and move out to friends and intimate others. As the teen's world becomes wider, adults in their lives continue to have influence on how the teens handle the rewards and struggles associated with social life.

In this chapter, you will learn to:

1. Discuss how teens develop socially
2. Analyze the roles of parents, peers, intimate relationships, and schools on social development
3. Describe the impact of violence, bullying, and teen dating violence on the social development of teens
4. Identify key focused interventions based upon learned concepts

SOCIAL DEVELOPMENT

The social or relational development of teens, like other forms of maturation, takes a predictable course with individual differences for each teen. Youth exert a lot of energy to become socially competent, and it is through varied experiences and processes of trial and error that teens learn to become social adults. All of this occurs within the contexts of their schools, homes, and communities. While learning to be empathic, sensitive to the needs of others, and relate to others socially, teens also learn about themselves and their strengths and areas of weakness. Developing a personal identity is often characterized and informed by bouncing ideas off of others and considering their insights. Social development is a product of nature and nurture and is characterized by selected processes, as found in Table 10.1.

TABLE 10.1 Processes of Social Development

Self-awareness	Understanding of one's personal traits, priorities, feelings, and responses to others.
Social awareness	Teens move from thinking as children, wherein everyone thinks like them or that emotions are universal or standard, to understanding reactions that are different from their own. Teens develop empathy to understand the feelings of others, read the emotions of others, see a situation from another point of view, and understand others' responses.
Social management	Teens learn to exercise emotional control by learning from role models and witnessing how emotions are handled. These lessons, and personal temperament, weave together to ensure that teens may monitor their emotions and responses to others. Self-regulation is a product of deliberate choices that override impulsive choices.
Developing friendships and relationships	Developing communication patterns, relationship boundaries, skills in conflict management, and methods to deal with peer pressure all inform how teens make and maintain friendships. The importance of peers throughout the life span warrant the considerable time, attention, and stress associated with the development of friendships and the skills needed to make and keep friends.

PARENTAL RELATIONSHIPS
AND INDEPENDENCE

Learning intimacy is a critical part of developing a personal identity and parents are the first intimate relationship that children develop—children are loved by parents in a close, honest, and caring relationship. Parental influence is a more powerful force on teens than race, income, and family structure combined in influencing health-related behaviors and decisions to engage in risky ones. The parental relationship allows children to learn to:

- Trust, express themselves, and learn about boundaries and support.
- Become independent from parents, make decisions, and take responsibilities for their own actions.
- Recognize and emulate stable emotional connections and predictable caretaking relationships.
- Handle difficult topics such as risk behaviors, sexual activity, and sensitive issues. Teens want to talk with parents but some teens claim that parents may not want to talk with them or that parents may be embarrassed or ill-equipped to handle such conversations.
- Adapt to personal and parental boundaries for behavior. Parameters on their behavior and others' expectations of them provide guidelines and denote that someone cares for them and their welfare. Boundaries that are too strict or do not allow for independent thoughts or actions may stifle a teen or cause rebellion. Research tells us that age-appropriate parental monitoring is associated with reduced risk behaviors and more positive outcomes on a wide spectrum of variables. Teens with adequate parental monitoring engage in fewer risky behaviors, have fewer pregnancies, are more successful in school, are less likely to engage in violence or fighting, and are physically healthier and engaged in health care than teens with less monitoring. As teens age they emulate health behaviors based on parental role modeling

and slowly take on increasing personal responsibility for health and decision-making.

Ongoing research examines the importance of two-parent families, the role of fathers, and the capacity for extended families in assisting with teens' social development. Creating a family identity, doing activities together, eating dinner together, and forming family bonds are protective factors against negative teen outcomes. Parenting styles influence family connectedness, a powerful force in teen lives, and are described in Table 10.2.

Parenting styles are associated with various outcomes with authoritative styles as most successful in American society. Teens with parents who are indifferent are noted to fare the worst. Parenting styles are culturally infused, and religion, ethnicity, and geography often dictate what style is considered most appropriate in a specific society. For example, some Asian communities contend that authoritarian parenting is preferable to other methods.

What about those teens without stable, capable, or available parents in their lives? As discussed previously, studies tell us that the presence of one positive role model is critical for success and achievement. Teens without such support in their family may seek adult role models in their schools, places of worship, or neighborhood. It is hoped that these are positive influences as teens develop their identities, sets of values, and decision-making patterns. One concern is that adults involved in crime are often able to identify teens without such ties and provide teens with consistent, loyal,

TABLE 10.2 Parenting Styles

Parenting Style	Warmth (Acceptance, Supportiveness, Responsiveness)	Boundaries (Demandingness, Expectations of Mature Behavior)
Authoritarian	Low	High
Indifferent	Low	Low
Authoritative	High	High
Indulgent	High	Low

and trusted adult guidance. Thus, teens may be lured into involvement in crime simply because of their need for adult engagement. To avoid this, we must try to foster parental abilities and, when not feasible, provide community supports to meet the needs of estranged and vulnerable youth.

PEERS AND RELATIONSHIPS

Friendships and sibling relationships lay down the groundwork for later intimate relationships. Although sometimes moving from parental to peer relationships is a conflict for families, this natural progression to reliance on friends is both healthy and constructive. As teens develop independence from parents, peers assist to:

- Serve as confidants, soundboards, and advisors.
- Pave the way for an intimate relationship with a significant other.
- Assist teens to develop positive self-esteem and mental health.
- Friend formation often occurs in a predictable pattern:
  - Early in adolescence, as in childhood, individuals tend to make friends who are similar to them in gender, interests, and other characteristics. This sexual cleavage, with a focus on same-sex friends, is thought to foster personal identity formation and self-esteem.
  - In middle adolescence, ages 14 to 16, teens become more tolerant of differences and make friends of both genders.
  - Older adolescents (17 and older) have more diversified groups of friends based on gender, associations, and interests such as those associated with work, home, and school. They also become increasingly interested in intimate relationships.
- The peer group is powerful throughout the life span and peers can have both positive and negative impacts on individuals.

Recent research demonstrates that teens engage in high-risk behaviors to a greater extent in the presence of peers. Allowing teens with and without friends to drive in a simulated car revealed that teens are more likely to succumb to riskier driving habits with peers in the car than when no peer was present. This difference was not sustained when adults were the drivers of the simulated cars.

- Young teens living in disadvantage, such as poverty, dysfunctional homes with decreased parental monitoring, or at-risk communities, were found to be more likely to take friends' advice about health and risk behaviors. These teens turned to friends for advice, role modeling, and resources, and were found to be more likely to engage in smoking tobacco, drinking alcohol, using marijuana, and sexual activity at earlier ages at the suggestion of their peers.

Sibling relationships are also important and serve as a "training ground" during the childhood and teen years. Table 10.3 discusses the characteristics of the sibling relationship.

TABLE 10.3 Unique Characteristics of the Sibling Relationship

Length	Entered in childhood and may be the longest relationship in a person's life
Tasks	Learn conflict management, empathy, and negotiating skills
Impact on health	May be as powerful as parental influence. Teens who smoke often report the impact of sibling influences
Parental monitoring	Sibling influence has been noted to be most powerful in those homes with decreased parental monitoring or capacity for parental support

The formation of intimate, romantic relationships with others is a focus of puberty and requires knowledge of self and an ability to let others in to see that self and appreciate its strengths and deficits. Dating has changed as the age of marriage has increased and the purposes of these romantic relationships may be different from the courtship and marriage known to the dating relationships of previous years. Dating is involved with learning about self and testing relationship skills with significant others. As teens learn about personal sexual responses and needs they also become interested in those of others. Surges in estrogen or testosterone allow for not only physical sexual development but also urges to explore sexuality. Preoccupation with sex, a rich fantasy world, and safe sexual behaviors are all "normal" and positive parts of the teen years. Dopamine is released when teens fall in love, oxytocin levels increase leading to feelings of nurturance and a desire for cuddling, and the body is well equipped to become sexually active. Culture, the media, and family values all impact intimate relationships and behaviors. It is the cognitive controls that are needed to make sure sexual relationships are safe, consensual, and engaged in with full knowledge. The intimate bonds formed during this period are the groundwork for future relationships and adulthood.

Despite previous research, newer studies reflect that boys and girls are equally invested in the intimacy of a relationship and value romance and caring. Girls tend to be involved with boys older than themselves, whereas boys tend to date girls the same age or younger. The shorter attention span of teens, changing priorities, and other developmental traits often predispose teens to shorter term relationships. Some newer research indicates that teens may have longer-term relationships but that these still may be in the minority of teen pairs. Relationships occur in phases, as noted in Table 10.4.

Break-ups of these relationships may be the cause of extreme distress. Teens often indicate that ending these intimate love affairs engenders feelings of depression, suicidal

TABLE 10.4 Phases of Relationships

Phase	Characteristics
Infatuation	Superficial relationships based on physical appearance, reputation, or beliefs, often short term, in which socializing and learning about self are the main tasks
Status	Establishment of relationships that go along with the needs of the peer group; individuals gain social status through relationships and attempt to gain approval from the group
Intimacy	Dominated by passion, preoccupation with the significant other, and elements associated with love and romance
Bonding	Characterized by commitment, love, long-term caring, discussion of the future, and assumptions of long-term connectedness

ideations, and withdrawal from those around them. Although adults may want to console and use a "this too shall pass" adage, it is important not to trivialize a sincere crisis in the teen's life.

FAST FACTS in a NUTSHELL

Current research analyzing the impact of very early dating found associations with increased mental health issues, incidences of depression, and early participation in intimate sexual activity without a development or understanding of the value of a meaningful or trusting relationship.

Teens and young adults may participate in gangs as part of their social interactions. Table 10.5 shares some characteristics of teen involvement in gangs.

TABLE 10.5 Teens and Gangs

Characteristics	Characterized by deviant behavior, name, and use of symbols such as colors, clothes, hand signs, tattoos, or jewelry
Involvement	Males in gangs tend to be involved in criminal activity, including drugs, alcohol, robbery, and violence. Girls who live at the periphery of gangs report high-risk sexual behaviors, drug and alcohol use, and participation in illegal acts
Functions	Researchers discuss that gang participation, for some teens, is a replacement for the intimacy and security missing in a dysfunctional home. Homes lacking in family life or parenting may predispose youth to seek out the camaraderie, belonging, and stability inherent to gang life. Teens may also be motivated to join gangs to earn money, as a result of peer pressure, for protection in unsafe schools and neighborhoods, and to gain status or respect.
Consequences	Concern over gangs is rooted in the impact on the individual and his or her potential future of crime, decreased school engagement, violence, and risk behaviors, and on the impact to the community. Gangs involved in criminal activities may instigate homicides, drug warfare, prostitution, and violent acts that serve to degrade and demoralize a neighborhood

SCHOOL CONNECTEDNESS

School is essentially a teen's "home away from home." More awake time is often spent at school than at home with family—teens spend about one third of their time at school. The influences of the school environment, teachers, and fellow students are powerful. School influences on teens are related to behaviors, values, and social development. Although the media and current events lead us to believe that schools are unsafe, the rate of school violence has actually declined since the early 1990s. Nonetheless, any violence in school must be addressed. Research tells us that individuals must feel safe in order to learn. Schools must be safe, comfortable, and stimulating to engage and keep students. Many schools institute safety measures including requiring visitors to sign in, metal detector checks, contraband sweeps, random dog sniffs, video surveillance, drug testing of athletes, and violence prevention programs.

School is one of the greatest forces, in addition to parents and peers, in influencing health risk behaviors. In addition to health teaching in the classroom, school nurses, wellness center staff, physical education teachers, health teachers, and athletic coaches provide education, role modeling, and access to care to attain and maintain health. Engagement in school, or school connectedness, is associated with better academic outcomes, higher academic performance, school completion, and decreased high-risk behaviors. Teens perceiving that teachers cared about them and were fair were found to be less likely to engage in risk behaviors.

The school dropout rate is a significant issue in American society, with the national average dropout rate of 12% and ranging from 10% to 50% in some school districts. The chance of earning a sustainable, legal wage in the United States without a high school diploma or its equivalency is not realistic in the current economy. This predisposes individuals to poverty, government subsidy dependence, and involvement in criminal activity. Dropping out is often the culmination of a variety of factors, including academic failure, undiagnosed learning disabilities, disciplinary measures, unintentional pregnancy, and the lure of a job. Strategies to keep teens in school need to re-engage learners, provide individualized interventions, and focus on technical educational routes to learn a valued trade.

VIOLENCE AND BULLYING

Violence

Violence and bullying are both forms of aggression that occur in adolescence, whether as victims, perpetrators, or witnesses. Violence is the threatened or actual use of physical force to cause actual or potential harm or emotional trauma.

Violence may be physical, verbal, or sexual and is a leading cause of death, disability, and injury in teens. Violence can be further differentiated as domestic, usually occurring in the home as in child or spousal abuse, or community violence, in which violence occurs outside the home and may occur between people who know or do not know each other. Violence can occur in the school, community, and home, taking a previously considered safe place and jeopardizing future feelings of security. Rates of violence have somewhat decreased in the past decades, as noted in Table 10.6.

Variables associated with violence include previous trauma, high levels of stress, peer pressure, drugs and alcohol, homelessness, mental health issues, availability of weapons, prejudice, poverty, lack of communication, adverse social conditions, and response to the media. Researchers attempted to find a correlation between violent videogames and the media, and the commission of violent acts. Although some scientists believe there is a strong relationship, others believe that video games are just another vehicle for witnessing violence, like movies, music, or books. To affirm this, one author made the assertion that violence rates are actually going down in the 10 years since video games have gained popularity.

Violence is thought to be transgenerational, with violence being passed down from parents to their children and subsequent generations. Learning to cope with and escape from violence is difficult and dealing with conflict using violent means is contagious and difficult to stop.

TABLE 10.6 Rates of Teen Violence

Youth Risk Behavior Survey Date	1991	2007	2011
Carried a weapon	26.1%	18%	16.6%
Carried a weapon on school property	7.3%	9.2%	7.4%
Carried a gun	7.9%	5.2%	5.1%
Had a physical fight	42.5%	31.5%	32.8%
Had a physical fight on school property	16.2%	12.4%	12%
Had property stolen or damaged	29.8%	27.1%	26.1%
Did not go to school for fear of safety	4.4%	5.5%	5.9%

FAST FACTS in a NUTSHELL

Homicide

- Homicide has remained the second- or third-highest cause of mortality in teens for the past several years
- Homicide is higher in males than females
- Homicide is highest in those aged 15 to 24
- Firearm homicides are increasing and represent the majority of homicides, 75% occurring with firearms found in the home
- 40% of homes with children have guns; in 25% of those homes, the guns are not under lock and key
- Rates of homicide are highest among Black and Hispanic youth

Bullying

Bullying is aggressive behavior that is intended to cause harm, occurs repeatedly, and exists where there is an imbalance of power. It is most common in the middle school years, with boys more involved than girls, and 30% of teens report that they were a victim or perpetrator of bullying. Additional research about bullying reveals:

- Boys tend to tease and hit, slap, or push. Girls tend to make fun of, create rumors, gossip, exclude others, and encourage others to reject individuals.
- Bullying may also be associated with differences in race, class, or other personal characteristics such as teens who are questioning their gender or sexual orientation, adding further torment to a difficult time in their lives.
- Although bullying has existed throughout time, there is a fear that with technology, increased access to weapons, and the more isolated nature of society, bullying has changed.

- Contrary to popular belief, most teens who are bullies are confident and have high self-esteem and are impulsive, aggressive, and popular but remain so based on power relationships.
- Bullies are at increased risk for delinquent and antisocial behavior later in life in addition to a higher rate of dropping out and mental health issues.
- Children who are bullied may be anxious, insecure, cautious, have low self-esteem, rarely defend themselves or retaliate, and lack social skills.
- Experts describe the "bystander" phenomenon, wherein youth witness bullying going on without acting.
- Parents may foster bullying behaviors, encouraging fighting and retaliation.

ABUSE AND TEEN DATING VIOLENCE

Domestic violence, including child, spousal, and elder abuse, all may impact the life of a teen. Contrary to popular belief, teens are abused at higher rates during adolescence. New or ongoing episodes of physical, emotional, and sexual abuse during the teen years gravely impact the teen's mental health, ability to function in school or home, and social skills. About 22% of all women and 7% of men experience intimate partner violence in their lifetime. Dating violence refers to physical, sexual, or psychological media for exerting power, violence between intimate partners during the teen years, and has gained the attention of parents, those working with teens, and policy makers. Although the data vary, Table 10.7 includes statistics related to teen dating violence (TDV).

Victims of TDV may have a history of family violence or child abuse and increased propensity to engage in high-risk behaviors. Perpetrators may demonstrate poor interpersonal skills, have a history of abuse or family violence, engage in high-risk behaviors, and have such personal traits as aggression, blaming, hostility, insecurity, jealousy, and dominance. In the short term, TDV may lead to injury, death, risky sexual behaviors, unhealthy dieting, substance use, suicidal

TABLE 10.7 Rates of Teen Dating Violence (TDV)

12% of high school students reported physical TDV

20% of high school students reported psychological TDV

10% of teens reported being hit, slapped, or physically hurt by a dating partner in the past year

9% of teens reported ending a relationship due to violence

8% of teen girls reported being forced to have sex against their will

21% of teen girls who are pregnant or parenting experienced TDV

TDV peaks in the 10th grade but may begin earlier

ideations, and physical fighting. In the long term, TDV may transfer to adult intimate partner violence, difficulties with relationships, and mental health issues.

Much of TDV occurs in secret and most cases are not reported. Victims may fear retaliation, feel loyalty toward their partner, feel at blame for the violence, or are embarrassed by the violent events. Violence may be "normalized" in their lives. Prevention efforts focus on the need for safe and expeditious means to report violence for victims, bystander education, and dealing with the fundamental issues of power, anger, and conflict management. Awareness of the issue and prevalence of TDV is often the launching point for school and community prevention programs. Teens with children experiencing TDV may have unique issues associated with children, economic dependence, loyalty, and the emotional ties of the children with the perpetrator.

Health care providers need to be on constant watch for TDV in each interaction with teens and be ready to assess for violence in teens' lives in any setting. Table 10.8 includes questions a health care provider may ask teens about TDV.

Following the assessment for violence in a relationship, referrals to counseling, resources, and shelters are critical to keep the teen safe. Believing the victim is integral allows the victim to feel supported and empowered to make difficult changes. Have ready a list of local referrals, including victim assistance programs, sexual assault shelters, and legal advocacy groups. Teen victims may not divulge issues, knowing

TABLE 10.8 Questions to Ask About TDV

Direct Questions

During the past year, did your boyfriend or girlfriend do anything physically to you that made you feel very uneasy or uncomfortable?

Do you feel safe at home? In your relationship?

Have threats of violence been made?

Does your partner seem jealous, controlling, or possessive?

Have you ever been forced to have sex?

Have weapons been used against you?

Probing Questions

Tell me about a time when you felt unsafe in your home

Tell me about a time when you felt unsafe in your relationship

To what type of violence have you been subjected?

Tell me about your partner's behaviors related to jealousy, control, or possessiveness

Tell me about your experiences when forced to have sex

Tell me about your experience when weapons were used against you

that any harm must be reported. Women at the age of majority have the choice to deny maltreatment, disclose information when ready, and to be aware that we as health care providers are concerned for their safety. Filing of protection or restraining orders, police involvement, and other procedures, though focused on victim safety, may be frightening and invasive, warranting sensitivity and caring by the health care provider. Reinforcing that the victim is innocent and that TDV is a crime may help teens move on with their lives.

FOCUSED INTERVENTIONS

- Empathy is a powerful means to allay violence, bullying, and interpersonal conflicts. Empathy-building strategies may be reinforced as individuals learn to consider others first. These may include:
  - Role modeling empathy, tolerance, and kindness.

- Involvement in service organizations to know and experience the needs of others.
- Cultivating hobbies and interests that enhance ideals about personal investment in things around them.
- Educating about realistic expectations of self and others.
- Having policies that reinforce and reward empathic behaviors.
- Reinforce caretaker and advocacy traits in teens to avoid idle bystander behaviors to bullying and violence. Speaking up, advocating for policies, and role modeling positive behaviors should be responsibilities of all teens.

- Reinforce conflict management strategies in interactions with peers and siblings.
  - Discuss that an individual's response is a choice: "You can't change the behavior of others, but you can change your response to them."
  - Assist teens to use stress management and "time-out" strategies.
  - Encourage teens to handle their emotions, use their developing prefrontal cortex, and address anger and conflict with means other than aggression and violence.
  - Foster decision-making and problem-solving skills at age-appropriate times.

- Provide teens with negotiating skills to help them in difficult situations. A strategy known as "invented dialogues" role-plays conflict situations and helps teens develop ready responses to requests or demands of others. If teens have these responses ready, they may use them in the event of a distressing situation.

- Teens who are of ethnic, racial, gender or sexual orientation, and religious minorities may be victims of bullying or live in communities plagued by violence. Advocates working with these youth have attempted to develop ethnic or minority pride among teens by focusing on the history, traditions, and aspects of their group that make them special. Also addressed were discrimination and the meaning of prejudice and racism. Teens strongly identifying with an ethnic or religious heritage have been found to have higher self-esteem, increased academic performance, a more defined sense of ethnic identity, and were less sensitive to racial discrimination.

- Coalitions from within neighborhoods, communities, and places of worship are powerful forces against aggression, bullying, and TDV. Health care providers may be part of coalition building, gathering stakeholders, and building advocacy skills with community partners.
- Health care providers may have an active role in creating environments where aggression (physical, verbal, or emotional) is not tolerated, bystander empowerment programs, and policies that encourage reporting of abuse, violence, and bullying.

SUGGESTED READING

Beal, A. C., Aisiello, J., & Perrin, J. M. (2001). Social influences on health-risk behaviors among minority middle school students. *Journal of Adolescent Health, 28,* 474–480.

DiClemente, R. J., Santelli, J. S., & Crosby, R. A. (Eds.). (2009). *Adolescent health: Understanding and preventing risk behaviors.* San Francisco, CA: Jossey-Bass.

Eaton, D. K., Kann, L., Kinchen, S., Shanklin, S., Flint, K. H., Hawkins, J., . . . Wechsler, H. (2012). Youth risk behavior surveillance—United States, 2011. *MMWR, 61*(4), 1–162.

Feinstein, S. (2007). *Teaching the at-risk teenage brain.* Lanham, MD: Rowman & Littlefield.

Herrman, J. (2005). The teen brain as a work in progress: Implications for pediatric nurses. *Pediatric Nursing, 31,* 144–148.

Herrman, J. W. (2009). There's a fine line . . . adolescent dating violence and prevention. *Pediatric Nursing, 35*(3), 165–170.

Herrman, J. W. (2010). Siblings' perceptions of diabetes and its management. *Journal of Pediatric Nursing, 25,* 428–437.

Herrman, J. W. (2013). How teen mothers describe dating violence. *Journal of Obstetric, Gynecologic, and Neonatal Nursing, 42,* 462–470.

Herrman, J. W., & Silverstein, J. (2012). Girls and violence: A review of the literature. *Journal of Community Health Nursing, 29*(2), 63–74.

Herrman, J. W., & Silverstein, J. (2012). Girls' perceptions of violence and prevention. *Journal of Community Health Nursing, 29*(2), 75–90.

McNeely, C., & Blanchard, J. (2009). *The teen years explained: A guide to healthy adolescent development.* Baltimore, MD: Johns Hopkins Bloomburg School of Public Health.

Ott, M. A., Rosenberg, J. G., McBride, K. R., & Woodcox, S. G. (2011). How do adolescents view health? Implications for state health policy. *Journal of Adolescent Health, 48*, 398–403.

Selekman, J., & Vessey, J. A. (2004). Bullying: It isn't what it used to be. *Pediatric Nursing, 30*(3), 246–249.

Serafini, T., Rye, B. J., & Drysdale, M. (Eds.). (2013). *Taking sides: Clashing views on adolescence.* New York, NY: McGraw-Hill.

Steinberg, L. (2008). *Adolescence.* New York, NY: McGraw-Hill.

Tasca, M., Zatz, M. S., & Rodriguez, N. (2012). Girls' experiences with violence: An analysis of violence against and by at-risk girls. *Violence Against Women, 18*(6), 672–680.

Yurgelun-Todd, D. (2003). *Frontline interview: Inside the teen brain.* Retrieved from http://www.pbs.org

SUGGESTED WEBSITES

Kids Health.Org
www.kidshealth.org/teen

Advocates for Youth
www.advocatesforyouth.org

The National Campaign to Prevent Teen and Unplanned Pregnancy
www.nationalcampaign.org

The Bureau For At-Risk Youth
www.at-risk.com

Office of Adolescent Health
www.hhs.gov/ash/oah

Teen Help.com
www.teenhelp.com

AddHealth
www.cpc.unc.edu/projects/addhealth

Centers for Disease Control and Prevention
www.cdc.gov/healthyyouth

The Urban Institute
www.urban.org

Healthy Teen Network
www.healthyteennetwork.org

Healthy People
www.healthypeople.gov

Johns Hopkins School of Public Health
www.jhsph.edu

Girl Scouts
www.girlscouts.org

The Search Institute
www.search-institute.org

Children's Hospital of Boston
www.childrenshospital.org

National Clearinghouse on Families and Youth
www.ncfy.acf.hhs.gov

Girls, Incorporated
www.girlsinc.org

Go Ask Alice
www.goaskalice.columbia.edu

Society for Adolescent Medicine and Health
www.adolescenthealth.org

The Dibble fund
www.dibblefund.org

University of Minnesota Extension
http://www1.extension.umn.edu/family/cyfc/our-services

Aspects of Caring for the Adolescent With Illness and Complex Health Issues

11

Acute and Chronic Illness

Although the adolescent years are characterized as healthier times, acute and chronic illnesses do impact teens. Teens deal with illness symptoms, management, and lifestyle changes. As teens transition to adulthood, the need to access adult health practitioners who have expertise in childhood chronic illnesses and how these diseases impact adult life must be considered.

In this chapter you, will learn to:

1. Discuss the impact of acute and chronic illness on teen health
2. Analyze the unique aspects of hospitalization when the client is a teen
3. Describe selected teen aspects associated with the management of asthma and diabetes
4. Identify key focused interventions based upon learned concepts

ILLNESS IN THE TEEN YEARS

Just as teens are unique individuals, so are their responses to acute or chronic illness. Illness is any condition that compromises one's ability to function and that requires specific medications, diet, medical technology, assistive devices, and/ or personal assistance. About 12% of teens have a chronic illness, or one where symptoms are present for greater than 1 year. Developmentally, teens are beginning to reason and understand abstract principles. This ability to comprehend things that they don't see or to understand processes that are complex enables them to understand such concepts as pain, internal cellular changes, and changes in health status. For some teens these concepts are not yet understood. This fact alone demands that each teen is assessed as an individual. Their level of understanding, ability to operationalize plans of care, and coping mechanisms need to be assessed. A lack of knowledge may lead to reduced compliance with the health care regimen or interpersonal conflicts between the teen and his or her caregivers. Their ability to cope with the changes demanded of this plan is critical to ongoing adjustment and adherence. Table 11.1 presents teens' concerns about chronic illness, as shared in focus groups.

As teens grow up they gain a greater sense of self-care and ability to become independent. They are beginning to understand their role in health practices and personal activities to keep healthy. Diagnosis with an acute or chronic illness may threaten these feelings of personal care. Teens may regress and expect parents to take care of them and attend to their treatment regimen. Additional concerns associated with chronic illness are found in Table 11.2.

Some illnesses require painful interventions, including blood draws, injections, dressing changes, exercises and physical therapy regimens, and diagnostic or surgical

---

TABLE 11.1 Teen Concerns About Illness

- Developing and maintaining friendships
- Being normal and getting on with life
- The importance of family
- The demands of treatment
- Experiences with school
- Relationships with health care professionals
- The future

Described by Taylor, Gibson, and Franck (2008).

TABLE 11.2 Other Concerns About Chronic Illness in Teens

- Decreased cognitive ability to understand and cope with illness
- Adherence to plan of care
- Independence, balancing personal and parental control
- Transition to adult practitioners
- Impact on school, activities, and peer relationships—threatened sense of personal mastery
- Quandary between personal and parental decision-making
- Symptom management—pain, immobility, treatments, diagnostics
- Rebellion and risk behavior

procedures. How teens deal with pain and discomfort is also very individual. Health care providers (HCPs) should use developmentally appropriate pain assessment techniques, measures to make care as atraumatic as possible, and involve teens in developing their own plan of care. Not only does that increase the teens' sense of control, but it also allows teens to understand "what is next" and their role in care.

FAST FACTS in a NUTSHELL

Atraumatic care is a new model of patient care in which measures are taken to reduce pain, restraint, and fear such as using intravenous access for as many medications as indicated, inserting long-term intravenous access devices, applying topical pain relief for invasive procedures, using age-appropriate and creative distraction techniques, enlisting the assistance of patients and families to provide restraint and immobilization, use of conscious sedation for procedures, and ensuring appropriate analgesia.

Education of teens includes comprehensive and honest teaching about the illness, symptoms, treatments, and potential outcomes. Teens need to have a thorough understanding of their medications including the therapeutic and side effects, specific instructions, and how to know the medications are working. Preparation for procedures should emphasize the sensory experiences associated with the test or invasive intervention. Teaching teens to anticipate the sights,

164

11. ACUTE AND CHRONIC ILLNESS

sounds, smells, and sensations will assist them to deal with the stress of diagnostics.

Depending on the physical nature of the illness, teens may be especially concerned about the impact on their appearance, their self-esteem, and the reactions of others. Loss of hair, apparatus, or symptoms that are visible may make the teen self-conscious about his or her illness. The illness may require them to "stand out" from peers and limit their social time. Frequent trips to the school nurse for medication, the need to eat a snack when others do not, or frequent absences may make the teen "look different" from their peers and call attention to his or her illness.

Teens who are medically fragile are perhaps the most vulnerable. Medically fragile is defined as those individuals who require medical technology and skilled care from parents, HCPs, and nurses on a daily basis. Ventilator dependency or the need for intravenous infusions, parenteral nutrition feeding routines, complex medication regimens, or physical care all contribute to medical fragility.

Just as conformity is a concern for all teens, the teen with an illness may feel that he or she is set apart from friends. Teens often seek "normalcy" in their lives. They may yearn for peer approval, be reluctant to talk about their illness, and feel frustration by the impact of chronic illness on the predictability of their future.

Acute and chronic illness may place stressors on the body that would make pregnancy or diagnosis with a sexually transmitted disease dangerous. An important component of illness management is to provide reproductive care and ensuring that birth control and condoms are used as protection. Genetic disorders or those that may be life-threatening in the event of a pregnancy warrant vigilant contraception and teaching. Other high-risk behaviors, including drugs, alcohol, smoking, or any that may potentially cause injury, need to be avoided and teens may need extra teaching to understand the implications of their actions. Some evidence reveals that teens with chronic illness engage in more risky behaviors than those without, indicating a target for instruction.

Optimal nutrition is required to meet the demands of adolescent growth patterns and to ensure healing or to cope with the stress of illness. Erratic or poor teen dietary habits, along with potential eating or gastrointestinal disorders, must also be addressed during an illness.

Parents may have unique concerns when their teen is diagnosed with or managing an illness. Juggling independence, regression, compliance, and rebellion offer unique challenges when a teen is ill. Increased demands on time, changes in responsibilities with siblings, financial concerns, and uneven responsibilities between parents may lead to discord. Stress will be accentuated when an illness has a poor prognosis, includes experimental or controversial treatments, or the course of illness is unknown. HCPs must provide support and referral to ensure optimal parental coping.

Teens with chronic or life-threatening illness may have an understanding of the potential of dying depending on their symptoms, the conversations they have had with family and caregivers, and their own knowledge about the illness and its course. Adolescents are beginning to have a better understanding of death as they mature, as noted in Table 11.3.

HCPs can do much to encourage honest and frequent conversations. Teens may resent the lack of communication, although well intentioned, that is done to protect them or to shelter them from information or choices. Whispered conversations, facial expressions of concern, and other tell-tale signs

TABLE 11.3 Adolescents' Conceptions of Death and Dying

- Beginning to understand the permanence of death
- As part of spiritual development, teens both adhere to and question parental or family beliefs about spirituality, religion, and death
- May exhibit egocentricity and may wish for death in retaliation for the wrongs of others, in a way inferring, "They'll be sorry when I am gone"
- The fear of the unknown or imagined consequences often exceed real issues associated with illness and death
- Most teens desire honest conversations about the trajectory of the illness, the potential outcomes, and the choices available during the course of illness and terminal stages of life
- Teens may understand palliative care but may require even more support than adults during end-of-life or hospice care

may suggest a situation worse than the truth. Teens deserve information and are ethically required to receive important information and to make choices to the extent required by law and family practices. Research tells us that teens want honesty and to participate in end-of-life decisions. HCPs should assess the individual teen's and the parent's levels of understanding of illness and adapt the discussion for their needs.

THE HOSPITALIZED ADOLESCENT

Hospitalization may be especially stressful for the adolescent. At a time when control and independence are paramount, hospitalization may take away these treasured elements. In addition, being away from peers and out of the daily routine of school or activities make teens feel like they are "missing something" and create a sense of loss. Although teens are seeking independence from parents, hospitalization may either limit this autonomy, creating feelings of resentment or sadness, or the adolescent may react with regressive behaviors. Parents and teens may be surprised by these reactions and need assistance to adapt to these responses.

Although hospitalization today is reserved for those who are truly ill, one of the greatest stressors of teens in hospitals is boredom. Table 11.4 provides some suggestions for easing the stress associated with hospitalization.

Because teens in hospitals may be especially fragile emotionally, it is important for HCPs to thoroughly assess clients' mental health status and repeat these assessments throughout the hospitalization. Research indicates that depression is common in teens with life-threatening and chronic illness. Counseling and management are especially important in hospitalized teens who lack the supports and comforts of home. Counselors with expertise in working with adolescents may best meet the needs of this population. Short-term medication management may be indicated to assist with coping during the hospitalization and drug interactions with current medications should be carefully avoided.

TABLE 11.4 Methods to Ease Teen Stress Related to Hospitalization

- Provide activities specific to the developmental level of teens, including school programming, child life, and special programs.
- Keeping up with school work or intellectual stimulation is also important during hospitalization. Communication between the teen's home school and agency staff is critical to ensure that the teen is current with school demands.
- Provide diversional activities to relieve boredom, encourage feelings of mastery, and distract from pain and other unpleasant symptoms.
- Provide bedside, age-appropriate activities such as crafts, videos, computer games, puzzles, art supplies, and board games.
- Teen rooms, equipped with music and low-effort games, away from younger children, are often found effective in "keeping teens busy" during a prolonged hospitalization.
- Explore leave policies that permit the patient to leave the hospital for important school or family events and return following their participation.
- Visitation policies to include asymptomatic friends, siblings, and family members enhance teens' moods and feelings of support.
- Agencies with pet visitation programs discovered the positive attributes and few negative issues associated with pets visiting with hospitalized teens.
- Encourage use of alternative modalities to enhance coping, including therapeutic touch, distraction, meditation, and others.

Active discharge planning, connecting to outpatient supports, and referral to community agencies allow for seamless care. Teens may be especially sensitive to disruptions in treatment or gaps in care. Communication to outpatient agencies about the teen's responses to treatment, individualized aspects of care, and unique characteristics of the teen will go far to enhance a smooth discharge to home.

DIABETES MELLITUS

More teens are being diagnosed with diabetes than ever before. Individuals must monitor their blood glucose levels and take insulin injections, along with monitoring nutritional glucose intake and exercise expenditures.

FAST FACTS in a NUTSHELL

There are a total of about 200,000 children and adolescents in the United States diagnosed with diabetes. 15,000 are diagnosed each year with type 1 diabetes. 4,000 are diagnosed each year with type 2 diabetes.

Knowledge of the signs and symptoms of hyperglycemia (high blood sugar) and hypoglycemia (low blood sugar) are needed on the part of the teen and the family in order to avoid life-threatening conditions. Table 11.5 describes the basics of diabetes mellitus.

Diabetes may be newly diagnosed during the teen years or may be an ongoing condition from a childhood diagnosis.

TABLE 11.5 Basics of Diabetes Mellitus (DM)

Type 1 DM

Cause	Multifactorial, potential genetic predisposition, viral insult, or stressful experience may precipitate symptoms
Pathophysiology	Absolute lack of insulin leading to unstable blood sugars and decreased glucose entering the cells of the body
Symptoms	Polyuria, polydipsia, polyphagia, weight loss, blurred vision, and fatigue; if the hyperglycemia progresses to ketosis, the patient may present with vomiting, ketotic breath, shortness of breath, and abdominal pain. Low blood sugar, from too much insulin, not enough carbohydrates, or exercise, may be manifested by fatigue, headache, sweatiness, tremors, irritability, visual changes, hunger, behavior changes, and changes in levels of consciousness.
Treatment	Capillary blood samples to assess blood sugar 6 to 12 times per day Doses of insulin adjusted per prescribed scales of dosages Insulin is administered via insulin syringe, insulin pen, or subcutaneous insulin pump inserted into the fatty layer of the skin and worn continuously

(continued)

Type 1 DM

Pumps provide a basal, or continuous dose, of insulin much like the human pancreas. They also allow for a bolus, or an extra dose, of insulin when the teen eats carbohydrates

More children and teens are being prescribed glargine (Lantus) insulin by injection. This formula of insulin does not peak in action so it offers patients a form of basal administration of insulin throughout the day

Adequate fluids are important to lower blood sugar and ensure hydration

Counting carbohydrates and using a carbohydrate-to-insulin ratio are important to calculate bolus amounts or meal dosages of insulin

Teens must also consider their level of exercise as they burn glucose to meet their energy needs and moderate their stress levels, since stress can raise the body's glucocorticoid levels. These stress hormones are glucose based and can raise blood glucose levels in response to stressful events

Type 2 DM

Causes	Obesity, poor nutrition, a sedentary lifestyle, and genetic factors
	Increased incidence of type 2 diabetes among minorities, including Hispanics, African Americans, Pacific Islanders, and American Natives
Pathophysiology	Characterized by relative lack of insulin
	May include cellular insulin resistance
Symptoms	May have no symptoms or may present with fatigue, polydipsia, or polyuria
	Manifestations unique to the individual
	Insulin resistance is associated with other health issues, including hypertension, hyperlipidemia, polycystic ovary disease, and acanthosis nigricans (hyperpigmentation of skin in select areas of the body)
Treatment	Focused on weight loss, portion control, exercise, and oral hypoglycemic agents (medications to lower blood sugar)
	May need insulin at times of illness or stress

Diagnosis as a young person suggests that the teen may live for many years with diabetes. Tight control of blood sugar, or keeping blood sugar within a narrow range, is recommended to reduce the potential of long-term complications to the cardiovascular, renal, visual, and nervous systems. Diabetes warrants a significant amount of discipline, control, and monitoring for any client. Some of these demands may be especially onerous for a teen.

- Diabetes requires a closely watched diet and timed eating. Although dietary restrictions have loosened in the past years, limiting simple carbohydrates and correlating meals with insulin administration are still needed. Teens often have less than optimal dietary habits and diabetes adds complexity to nutrition planning and monitoring.
- Tight control of diabetes avoids long-term complications. As discussed, teens may not appreciate the need to control today's behavior to avoid issues in the future. The need to focus on immediate and relevant complications is helpful here.
- Insulins have different onsets, peaks, and durations and are prescribed to meet the individual needs of the teen. This may lead to confusion and requires thorough teaching.
- Teens, especially girls, learn that omitting doses of insulin can lead to "quick weight loss." Unfortunately, high blood sugars without control can lead to diabetes ketoacidosis and hospitalization. Education is critical to avoid life-threatening conditions.
- Drinking alcohol may be especially complex for the teen with diabetes. Although abstaining from alcohol is the best choice, teens often drink with the belief that alcohol drinks have carbohydrates. Ingesting alcohol actually suppresses liver function and the ability to break down glycogen to glucose when blood sugar falls. Teens may experience significant lows, often mistaken for or in addition to intoxication, when drinking alcohol. An important recommendation is to eat a protein-filled meal prior to drinking to avoid hypoglycemia.
- As teens become more independent in their blood sugar control they often manage their own highs and lows.

Because some teens suffer from hypoglycemia unawareness, teaching should be directed toward the differentiation of high and low blood sugar levels and helping the teen tune into his or her individual symptoms. Family members and friends should also be apprised of these symptoms.

- Sick-day care is an important aspect of teens' managing their blood sugar levels. Teens often feel that if they are not eating they don't need to take insulin. Again, stress hormone secretion raises blood sugar and is one of the leading precursors to diabetic ketoacidosis, requiring narrow control of blood sugar levels.

ASTHMA

More children and teens are diagnosed with asthma than ever before. Comorbidity with allergies and an increasing number of allergenic agents, in addition to questions about air quality, cleanliness, and other triggers (aggravating agents), have led to significant research about the current causes and management of asthma. Teens may be diagnosed during their childhood or newly diagnosed during adolescence.

=======FAST FACTS in a NUTSHELL

Asthma is the most common childhood illness.

9.5 million children or 20.9% of high school students have been diagnosed with asthma.

6.7 million children or 10.9% of high school students are currently being treated for asthma.

Asthma generates: 7 million outpatient visits, 754,000 emergency department visits, and 200,000 hospitalizations annually, with an increase in hospitalizations of 225% in the past 30 years.

Costs associated with asthma care exceed $19.7 billion annually.

Asthma is the No. 1 reason for school absenteeism.

TABLE 11.6 Basics of Asthma

Pathophysiology	Narrowing of the airways (bronchoconstriction), edema of the airways, excessive mucus production
Causes	Genetic predisposition and environmental
Symptoms	Shortness of breath, coughing, wheezing, increased work of breathing, lower oxygen saturation levels, and reduced peak flow readings (assessing the amount of air exhaled and providing a quantitative measure of the air moved through the lungs)
Treatment	Inhalers that deliver bronchodilators, steroids, antihistamines, expectorants, and other medications to the lower airways to open them, reduce edema, and loosen mucus. At times, oral medications are also prescribed to enhance airway dilation or to reduce histamine responses in the body

Asthma comes in different forms (Table 11.6). When related to a concurrent viral or bacterial illness, reactive airway disease may be managed with treatment of the illness in addition to symptomatic treatment. Exercise-induced asthma may be related to exertion and may require only episodic care during specific times. Classic asthma includes remissions and exacerbations in response to individual client triggers. Each client is instructed to identify, and potentially avoid, these triggers. These may include molds, dust, animal dander, pollen, exertion, allergenic substances, smoke, emotional stress, and others.

Asthma, like diabetes, is a life-threatening chronic condition and may include acute exacerbations. As the teen matures and possibly becomes more responsible for treatment, important considerations include:

- Patients are often prescribed several treatment regimens based on their symptoms, progressing from a parent-managed to teen-managed regimen. As teens learn about their treatment they should be allowed the independence, with surveillance, to make decisions about the correct inhaler to use. As teens gain knowledge about their disease and understand its management, they learn to deal with the use of the inhalers, to take their own peak flow readings, and to avoid triggers.

- Inhalers have specific procedures to ensure safe administration of medications and require careful, device-specific teaching.
- Patients are often ordered a "preventer" inhaler or set of medications that are administered daily as prophylaxis against asthmatic symptoms. They are also given a "rescue" regimen to be used during acute symptoms. If taken when not really needed, the body may become tolerant to the rescue medication's effects. This could lead to ineffectiveness of the rescue medication when it is most needed and is associated with asthma-related mortality.
- Emotional triggers in asthma can become tricky during the teen years. Although all asthmatic symptoms should be taken very seriously, thorough assessments must be conducted to ensure the validity of the symptoms and to avoid erroneous treatment. Individual and family counseling are sometimes indicated if these issues become out of control during the teen years.
- Because exacerbations of asthma may be related to viral or bacterial illnesses, we must ensure that teens avoid illness, including getting adequate rest, optimal nutrition and hydration, avoiding ill persons when possible, and good handwashing techniques.
- Teens may often misread the gravity of these symptoms. Inaccurate perceptions of asthma symptoms lead to increased hospitalization, emergency department visits, and school absences. This warrants teen-specific education on symptoms that indicate a need for treatment.
- Few teen-specific educational programs exist to address asthma. New web-based programs, group discussions, asthma camps, clinic-based interventions, and other unique teaching strategies are emerging to meet this need.

FOCUSED INTERVENTIONS

- Establish behavioral contracts with teens who are ill or hospitalized. Set up ground rules and plans of care encouraging mutual collaboration and knowledge of consequences. Have teens be part of the plan such that they feel invested in its success, understand the positive and negative consequences of actions, and are invested in the outcomes.

- An important element of family-centered care is to ensure that the entire family (siblings, parents, and extended members) has a good understanding of the illness, hospitalization, and course of events. Siblings' needs must be assessed for developmental understanding of the issues associated with the status of the teen and for their personal role. This may include a change in their own lives, routines, or activities; a more active set of responsibilities within the home or with the ill sibling; and a change in family dynamics.

- Screening, early diagnosis, and rapid treatment are associated with the most positive outcomes in teens. This validates ongoing physical examinations and health surveillance during the teen years.

- Ongoing research assesses teens' abilities to self-manage illnesses within the school environment. The ability to carry inhalers, insulin, blood glucose monitors, and glucose sources in school, to sports practices, and during school activities is controversial but is gaining increased support. Allowing teens to rapidly treat their health changes may be associated with better outcomes and fewer complications.

- Smoking is discouraged in all teens. For teens with asthma it is associated with exacerbation of symptoms and causes increased risk of cardiovascular disease in teens with diabetes.

- An important component of care is determining teen and parent level of decision-making. Some prefer the more paternalistic model of being "told what to do" while others want an active, shared role in all decisions. HCPs may assess the level of information a family prefers and individualize care accordingly.

- Most importantly, for teens with chronic or acute illness it is paramount to treat the person, not the illness.

Buckner, E. B., Simmons, S., Brakefield, J. A., Hawkins, A. K., Feeley, C., Frissell Kilgore, L. A., . . . Gibson, L. (2007). Maturing responsibility in young teens participating in asthma camp: Adaptive mechanisms and outcomes. *Journal for Specialists in Pediatric Nursing, 12*(1), 24–36.

Chase, H. R. (2002). *Understanding diabetes* (10th ed.).Denver, CO: Barbara Davis Center for Childhood Diabetes.

Herrman, J. W. (2006). Listening to children's voices: Perceptions of the costs and rewards of diabetes and its treatment. *Journal of Pediatric Nursing, 21*(3), 211–221.

Herrman, J. W. (2010). Siblings' perceptions of diabetes and its management. *Journal of Pediatric Nursing, 25*, 428–437.

Joseph, C., Ownby, D. R., Havstad, S. L., Saltzgaber, J., Considine, S., Johnson, D., . . . Johnson, C. C. (2013). Evaluation of a web-based asthma management intervention program for urban teenagers: Reaching the hard to reach. *Journal of Adolescent Health, 52*, 419–426.

Kaufman, F. R., Gallivan, J. M., & Warren-Boulton, E. (2009). Overview of diabetes in children and teens. *American Journal of Health Education, 40*(5), 259–263.

Knopf, J. M., Hormung, R. W., Slap, G. B., DeVellis, R. F., & Britto, M. T. (2008). Views of treatment decision-making from adolescents with chronic illnesses and their parents: A pilot study. *Health Expectations, 11*, 343–354.

Lewandowski, L., & Telser, M. D. (Eds.). (2003). *Family centered care: Putting it into action.* Silver Spring, MD: American Nurses Association/Society of Pediatric Nurses.

Lyon, M. E., McCabe, M. A., Patel, K. M., & D'Angelo, L. (2004). What do adolescents want? An exploratory study regarding end of life decision-making. *Journal of Adolescent Health, 35*(529), e1-529–e6-529.

McNeely, C., & Blanchard, J. (2009). *The teen years explained: A guide to healthy adolescent development.* Baltimore, MD: Johns Hopkins Bloomburg School of Public Health.

Rhee, H., Belyea, M. J., & Halterman, J. S. (2011). Adolescents' perception of asthma symptoms and health care utilization. *Journal of Pediatric Healthcare, 25*(2), 105–113.

Sawyer, S. M., Drew, S., Yea, M., & Britto, M. T. (2007). Adolescents with a chronic condition: Challenges living, challenges treating. *The Lancet, 369*, 1481–1489.

Sharpe, D., & Rossiter, L. (2002). Siblings' perceptions of children with chronic illness: A meta-analysis. *Journal of Pediatric Psychology, 27,* 699–711.

Spratling, R., & Weaver, S. R. (2012). Theoretical perspective: Resilience in medically fragile adolescents. *Research and Theory for Nursing Practice, 26*(1), 54–68.

Srof, B., Taboas, P., & Velsor-Friedrich, B. (2011). Adolescent asthma education programs for teens: Review and summary. *Journal of Pediatric Health Care, 26*(6), 418–426.

Srof, B., Velsor-Friedrich, B., & Penckofer, S. (2011). The effects of coping skills training among teens with asthma. *Western Journal of Nursing Research, 34,* 1043–1061.

Taylor, R. M., Gibson, F., & Franck, L. S. (2008). The experience of living with a chronic illness during adolescence: A critical review of the literature. *Journal of Clinical Nursing, 17,* 3083–3091.

Velsor-Friedrich, B., Vlasses, F., Moberly, J., & Coover, L. (2004). Talking with teens about asthma management. *The Journal of School Nursing, 20*(3), 140–148.

SUGGESTED WEBSITES

Kids Health.Org
www.kidshealth.org/teen

The Bureau For At-Risk Youth
www.at-risk.com

Society for Adolescent Medicine
and Health
www.adolescenthealth.org

Healthy People
www.healthypeople.gov

Johns Hopkins School of
Public Health
www.jhsph.edu

Learn to Be Healthy
www.learntobehealthy.org/
teens

Office of Adolescent Health
www.hhs.gov/ash/oah

Children's Hospital of Boston
www.childrenshospital.org

University of Minnesota
Extension
http://www1.extension.umn.
edu/family/cyfc/our-services

12

Technology and Teen Health

Technology is an important asset in enhancing health. It also offers some challenges and unique issues with regard to teens. Newer concepts like cyberbullying, sexting, tweeting, and social media often change the landscape of adult–teen relationships and may create unsafe situations for teens and adults. This chapter introduces and clarifies the role of adult caregivers and health care providers related to teens and technology.

In this chapter, you will learn to:

1. Discuss how teens engage in and use technology
2. Explain the role of technology in positively and negatively influencing teen health
3. Analyze behaviors associated with cyberbullying
4. Identify key focused interventions based upon learned concepts

TECHNOLOGY AND TEENS

Technology may have both positive and negative effects on teen health. If you ask many teens, technology is not a separate entity but is instead part of their daily lives. Using their phone to wake up in the morning, check the weather, text friends, answer questions, take pictures, listen to music, access social media, complete homework, find directions, purchase items, play games with people around the world, and sustain relationships are just samples of how teens use and depend upon technology. Books are replaced by search engines, online and hardcopy graphic novels, graphic novellas, telenovellas, and audio libraries. Teens may now hold the world in the palm of their hand, and important interventions are evolving to address this. Specially designed websites and mobile platforms exist to teach about safe sexual behavior, the importance of a designated driver, the hazards of smoking, and assessing your daily nutritional intake against recommended guidelines. Health professionals are using e-mail, texting, social media, and video chatting to connect with clients, provide education, communicate test results, and keep clients informed of health care regimen changes. It is thought that this electronic communication saves time, ensures client partnering in care, and ends frustrating wait times. These forms of communication, however, raise issues about confidentiality and adherence to the Health Care Portability and Affordability Act (HIPAA).

FAST FACTS in a NUTSHELL

Cell Phone

- 75% of teens own a cell phone
- 54% of teens use their cell phone for texting
- 24% of teens use their cell phone for instant messaging
- 25% of teens use their cell phone for social network access

Computers allow teens to connect, talk, interact with others in games and puzzles, and engage in social media for business and leisure purposes. Satellite map sites allow us to see our destinations while we get directions. Electronic bulletin boards allow us to plan events, get ideas, and share with others. Search engines answer our questions, provide us with recipes, help us do our errands, and meet myriad informational needs. This broadening world expands our reach, access to information, and how we function day to day. Electronic resources have been especially valuable for those with chronic illness, those who may be isolated related to the demands of their disease, or those seeking support or camaraderie with others in the same situation. Blogs, websites, social networking sites, and discussion board sites may be extremely valuable as a teen deals with the rigors of an illness, trauma, or treatment. Many believe that social network sites are positively associated with self-expression, social capital formation, and the ability to develop a personal identity. Adults and teens alike find social media to be a way to meet people with common interests, send and receive pictures and videos, keep in contact with friends at a distance, relate to others, and keep connected with current events. Social networking sites (Facebook, MySpace, Instagram, and Twitter), dating sites (MyLOL.net), gaming sites (Club Penguin, Second Life, and the Sims), video sites (YouTube), chat rooms, and blogs all provide forums for teens to explore, interact, and socialize.

FAST FACTS in a NUTSHELL

Computers and Internet

- 86% of teen homes have a computer
- 75% of teen homes have Internet access
- 90% of teens use the Internet daily
- 70% of teens have a social network site
- More than 50% of teens log into their favorite social network site at least one time per day and 22% log in 10 times per day
- 30% of teens send nude or seminude photos over the Internet or via text on their phone
- 54% of postings on social media sites discuss risky behavior (smoking, drinking alcohol, sexual behavior, violence, and drugs)
- 12% of teens with Facebook accounts admit their parents are unaware of the account
- Most online sexual predators are adult men luring teens who are 12 to 17 years of age

TECHNOLOGY AND THREATS TO TEEN HEALTH

As with most positives, there are downsides to this technology evolution as well. Part of the issue with technology is the rapid rate of growth and change in what is available, often leaving parents and adults always "a few steps behind" in their development. Concern has emerged as teens spend less time in actual social interactions and more time in these virtual relationships. Some adults are worried that the development of interpersonal skills, the ability to work with others and in teams, and reading of nonverbal cues may be lost with the explosion of these electronic methods. Others contend that these media interfaces are the social interaction platforms of tomorrow and are cultivating critical skills for adulthood. Social media and virtual resources are important ways to reach and engage teens, and many feel prevention efforts need to focus on these routes to reach today's teens. Characteristics of the teen years, including developing decision-making skills, self-regulation, dealing with peer pressure, and addressing conflict, may require a level of adult monitoring and assistance as teens mature. Because social media is largely unmonitored, there may be times that teens are placed at risk.

Teens may be victims of stalking, predators, accessing pornography, or other inappropriate activities related to Internet access. Identified issues such as "Facebook depression" (in which teens seek out social and emotional approval from their social networking sites and may experience sadness, anxiety, withdrawal from daily life, and suicidal ideations from overreliance on their virtual world), issues with sexting, clique formation, cyberbullying, Internet addiction, and sleep deprivation have emerged as a result of the social media explosion. Teens may also not understand the impact on the "digital footprint" of potentially impulsive actions, such as sending provocative photographs or sexually explicit materials via the Internet. States and schools have responded to sexting issues by developing laws and policies to assist in curtailing these activities. The permanency and transferability of information and the potential to go "viral"

TABLE 12.1 Cyberbullying Data

42% of teens report being bullied online

19% of teens report harassment online or cyberbullying

21% of teens received a threatening message online

38% of teens know someone who was a victim of cyberbullying

More than one third of those who were cyberbullied also reported live bullying in their school or community

Boys and girls both participate in cyberbullying; girls are most likely to be victims

58% of those teens who experienced or witnessed cyberbullying did not report it to an adult

over the Internet may be incomprehensible for teens but may have long-reaching implications for their safety, professional lives, and personal privacy (Table 12.1).

Cyberbullying is defined as repeated and intentional harm inflicted through electronic text. These behaviors may subjugate the teen based on race, sexual orientation, or personal identity and may be demeaning, cruel, or violent. Types of cyberbullying are cited in Table 12.2.

"Flame wars" are concerted online bullying attacks that escalate and lead to ostracizing the individual, chasing him

TABLE 12.2 Methods of Cyberbullying

Instant messaging—negative messages, death threats	Developing websites with insulting or other information
"Blowing up the phone" with many messages	Internet polling
"Warning wars"	Impersonation of others
Stealing passwords—change profile or lock out of account	Gaming and cheating in another person's name or stalking with game sites
Comments on blogs—damage reputation or divulge information on others	Sending malicious codes, malware, or viruses; hacking
Signing someone up for junk or other unsolicited mail	Sending pictures or pornography—locker room, bathroom, or dressing room pictures

or her off the website, or public embarrassment. One difference of cyberbullying, in contrast to in-person bullying, is that it may be more difficult to escape. It is also more pervasive, difficult to track, anonymous, and can be more public such that the effects are more significant.

While the web, social networking, and technology are no longer something that can be taken from a teen's life, characteristics of youth and brain development warrant surveillance and supervision by caring adults. The focused interventions for this chapter include several expert suggestions to enhance the health of teens related to technology.

FOCUSED INTERVENTIONS

- Do not allow computers in the bedroom. Keep the bedroom a place for sleep. This encourages family time and discourages constant access to the computer. This may be obsolete in teens who rely on their cell phones for social media. Household rules and boundaries may address these issues. Some experts advise developing ground rules on time spent on phones and computers, rather than focusing on the place or location in the house, to address this issue.
- Teach teens about Internet stalking and their vulnerability to predators. Emphasize the need to keep personal information off the Internet.
- Use adult controls but also monitor time on the Internet. Many teens are able to circumvent controls, enhancing their vulnerability.
- If cyberbullying is taking place, try to shut down the site or blog. Encourage teens not to respond to online bullying.
- Parents may "Friend" teens on social networks and educate themselves on technology and social networks available.
- Open and honest discussion about privacy and the "digital footprint" are important and may be engaged

in several times as the teen develops. Have discussions about unhealthy, harmful, or inappropriate messaging.

- Discuss issues such as stalking, cyberbullying, and predators in open, honest, and realistic ways.
- Ensure that teens are aware that everything on the Internet is not true, valid, vetted, or based on sound principles. Being an informed and wary consumer of information is critical to accessing web-based content and may have significant health impacts.
- Monitor teens' activities, especially if Internet friendships evolve to become in-person meetings. Research indicates that 75% of those teens who have live contact with individuals they met online do so more than once. Teens need information about adult predators and the inappropriate nature of adult–teen meetings.

SUGGESTED READING

Herrman, J. (2005). The teen brain as a work in progress: Implications for pediatric nurses. *Pediatric Nursing, 31*, 144–148.

Jacobs, H., & Popick, R. (2012). Utilization of internet resources for adolescents coping with chronic conditions. *Pediatric Nursing, 38*(4), 228–233.

McBride, D. L. (2011). Risks and benefits of social media for children and adults. *Journal of Pediatric Nursing, 26*, 498–499.

McNeely, C., & Blanchard, J. (2009). *The teen years explained: A guide to healthy adolescent development*. Baltimore, MD: Johns Hopkins Bloomburg School of Public Health.

Serafini, T., Rye, B. J., & Drysdale, M. (Eds.). (2013). *Taking sides: Clashing views on adolescence*. New York, NY: McGraw-Hill.

Steinberg, L. (2008). *Adolescence*. New York, NY: McGraw-Hill.

Woolford, S., Blake, N., & Clark, S. J. (2013). Texting, tweeting, and talking: E-communicating with adolescents in primary care. *Contemporary Pediatrics, 30*(6), 12–18.

Zazik, M. A. P., Manasse, S. M., & Orrell-Valente, J. K. (2012). Adolescents' self-presentation on a teen dating web site: A risk content analysis. *Journal of Adolescent Health, 50*, 517–520.

SUGGESTED WEBSITES

Advocates for Youth
   www.advocatesforyouth.org
The National Campaign
   to Prevent Teen and
   Unplanned Pregnancy
   www.nationalcampaign.org
The Bureau For At-Risk Youth
   www.at-risk.com

Girls, Incorporated
   www.girlsinc.org
Johns Hopkins School of
   Public Health
   www.jhsph.edu
Society for Adolescent
   Medicine and Health
   www.adolescenthealth.org

13

Ethics, Marginalization, and Advocacy

This text has reinforced the wonderful, and complex, nature of today's teens. As teenagers navigate their way to adulthood they confront challenges and issues. This chapter addresses ethical issues important to consider with teens, the marginalization of teens in today's society, and global issues related to adolescents. In closing, the chapter charges readers to serve as advocates for teen health.

In this chapter, you will learn to:

1. Explore ethical issues unique to the teen years
2. Analyze how teens are marginalized in today's society
3. Discuss how teens are viewed around the world and the global state of teen health
4. Identify key focused interventions based upon learned concepts

ETHICS

Health care providers (HCPs) frequently confront ethical issues in practice and may be skilled at dealing with them on a professional basis. When adolescents are added to the equation these issues may become a little more complex. An adolescent's abilities to consent to health care, participate in research, access preventive health information, and other areas confronted within the health care environment are largely dictated by state laws or policies and are designed to protect the adolescent. These protections, though, may reflect how society views teens and may differ based on state and local policies. Table 13.1 includes some key terms addressing teen rights.

Consent for health treatment, choices about refusal of treatment, and areas of consent in which parents or guardians and teens differ in opinion may be confronted during patient care and offer challenges to the HCP. Adolescent participation in experimental therapies, solicitation of mental health services, and adherence to a plan of care may offer

TABLE 13.1 Legal Definitions Regarding Teens

Age of majority	When a teen is considered an adult 18 years in most states Four states use 19 or 21 years In some states, age of majority differs from the age of consent
Age of consent	Age when an individual may be able to consent to or give permission for invasive or surgical procedures, health care, research studies, activities, access to services, and other resources. May be dictated by state law or agency policy
Minors	Less than the age of majority Generally requires permission consent from parents or appointed guardians and may require assent from teens
Mature minors	State law dictates that these teens receive more rights than a child, but less than an adult
Emancipated minors	Affords youth additional rights May be emancipated by participation in the military, parenting a child, documented self-sufficiency and living independent of parents, marriage, or graduation from high school. Many states use a legal, court-directed process of emancipation known as the Judicial Bypass Mechanism. Some states do not have mature minor or emancipation stipulations or laws, so each case must be addressed by the courts on an individual basis

All states allow for adolescents to consent for routine treatments without parental consent, but the limitations and specifics of these policies vary from state to state. These policies may reflect local beliefs on adolescent cognitive and decision-making abilities and on adult perceptions of the health needs of youth.

ethical dilemmas with regard to the care of teens. Some practitioners caution that teens may not seek out health care for sensitive or private health issues due to the need to solicit parental consent for treatment. The most debated ethical dilemmas related to youth are the laws, policies, and issues associated with reproductive health and risk behaviors. Table 13.2 discusses selected controversial areas related to adolescent health education and services.

Research is an important area in which teens are offered a level of protection and HCPs may need to provide advocacy for patients. Dependent upon the level of risk associated with the research, teens must have one or both parents' permission in order to participate in research and must provide personal assent in order to meet institutional review board standards. Unfortunately, until recently, the reluctance to place children and adolescents at risk has limited the depth of research and findings available about those age groups. Authors assert that teens would benefit from greater involvement in the consent process to enhance autonomy and personal responsibility for actions and that parent-focused permission processes may marginalize teens.

The confidentiality afforded health care may also depend upon federal and state laws and policies, such as the Health Insurance Portability and Accountability Act (HIPAA) Privacy Rule, in addition to agency practices. HIPAA launched protections but also raised concerns for teens. Passed in 2002, HIPAA protects the privacy of individual's health information and medical records. Although confidentiality has been a long-standing principle in health care, infractions

TABLE 13.2 Controversial Areas Related to Adolescent Health Education and Services

Area of Controversy	Examples
Drugs and alcohol	
Education	Teaching about types of drugs and other substances
Services	Needle exchange programs Treatment for addiction to substances without parental consent Consent for education, testing, and treatment for HIV
Sexual health	
Education	Abstinence-only versus comprehensive sexuality education Safe sexual behavior education Age of consensual sexual relationships Information related to sexual orientation and gender identity
Services	Condom distribution Prescribing contraception without parental consent Abortion services (consent needed from parents, consent needed from father, and waiting periods all vary by state) Access to prenatal services Consent for education, testing, and treatment for HIV and sexually transmitted infections Age of sexual partners and access to treatment
Abuse	
Laws	Mandatory reporting laws for minors, mature minors, and emancipated minors related to child abuse, neglect, dependency, unlawful sexual contact, and threat to harm self or others Age of sexual partners/statutory rape laws Child support laws and enforcement

occurred. In addition, technology, the electronic health record, and the Internet offer greater potential for breaching confidentiality. This ruling ensures confidentiality of health care provision to teens, but also represents a conflicting ideology of parental rights to information and confidentiality information associated with health care payments. One of the leading reasons teens do not seek out care is lack of privacy and the potential for parental notification. States, schools, and HCPs differ on their interpretations of the HIPAA privacy stipulations as they relate to reproductive care, abortions, treatment for substance use and abuse, and mental health care. Future interpretations or changes to HIPAA may clarify the rights held by teens, parents, and guardians.

MARGINALIZED YOUTH

Teens are often thought to be moderately marginalized in society because of their potential lack of voice, circumstances, and experiences. Age is one area of marginalization and may coincide with poverty, ethnicity, race, sexual or gender orientation, or gender inequities. Some consider the teen years an inherently disempowered age cohort, referring to teens are "second-class citizens." Due to their dependency on adults, their age-related cognitive limitations, and their lack of independent resources, some may consider teens as having less value. Others consider teens a critical force in society, the important next generation, and the creative and enthusiastic hope for tomorrow.

Most teens are protected by their parents, other adults, and the child welfare rules, laws, and regulations. There are some teens who are more vulnerable due to their social circumstances, including those who live in poverty, who are foster children or children of incarcerated parents, runaways, teens who are homeless, teens who are incarcerated, teens in out-of-home care, and teens with tenuous home lives. Teens living in poverty have a greater risk of chronic illness, higher rates of hospitalization, more traumatic injuries and deaths, nutrition deficits, and higher incidences of infectious diseases, homelessness, and educational or occupational challenges. Researchers tell us that teens in poverty are exposed to fewer experiences; their brains have fewer opportunities for pruning, and, therefore, they may process information and learn slower than individuals who are more fortunate.

Teens focused on safety and survival are already thought to learn less due to stress and its impact on the hippocampus. Teens who are disadvantaged may be disempowered by their lack of a voice in their destiny and have fewer choices in the directions of their future, increasing their potential to engage in high-risk behaviors. These teens are those most in need of adult advocacy and our investment as concerned HCPs!

TEENS AROUND THE WORLD: THE UNITED NATIONS FOCUS ON ADOLESCENCE

As defined in Chapter 1, the period of adolescence is socially constructed and defined by the context. Adolescence is framed differently around the world, and race, gender, age, religion, and other characteristics further inform how adolescents are perceived by a society.

Although the health of teens in the United States has been the focus of this text and we have highlighted several threats to teen health, teens fare very well in the United States compared to other countries. The World Health Organization (WHO), the United Nations agency in charge of global health, developed eight Millennium Development Goals (MDGs) related to population health. These are found in Table 13.3.

Although all of these goals may be applied to the teen years, select ones may be highlighted. Reducing child mortality is an

---

TABLE 13.3 WHO/UN Millennium Development Goals

1	Eradicate extreme hunger and poverty
2	Achieve universal primary education
3	Promote gender equality and empower women
4	Reduce child mortality
5	Improve maternal health
6	Combat HIV/AIDS, malaria, and other diseases
7	Ensure environmental sustainability
8	Develop a global partnership for development

important worldwide goal, with child mortality being higher in infancy and early childhood than during the adolescent years. Nonetheless, teen mortality is an issue related to communicable illnesses, including AIDS, and lack of resources, starvation, a dearth of potable water, lack of medical care, lack of immunizations, and decreased access to treatment. Improving maternal health is important for both rearing of healthy teens but also for teen mothers. In many developing nations the average age of motherhood is lower than that in the United States. Different roles of women, gender and socioeconomic inequities, resources, and health care access all influence how teen mothers may fare in the antenatal period. Access to prenatal care, educated health care practitioners, including midwives, and encouragement of breastfeeding are all strategies designed to promote positive health outcomes. HIV is a severe threat around the world and prominent among teens. Access to medications, education and supplies to ensure safe sexual practices, drug use prevention, and safe needles may reduce the devastation posed by HIV worldwide.

FOCUSED INTERVENTIONS

- Although teens may be a verbal cohort in our society, the fact remains that "teens don't vote!" Teens need our advocacy and our voices to ensure their needs are considered in today's political and economic environment. Reinforcing that teens are the next productive generation and will care and provide for today's current earning generation is a critical platform upon which to build advocacy efforts.
- Although teens may need representation by the adults in their world, their own voices need to be heard! Research, programing, and policies need to capture teens' own thoughts, advisory councils need teen membership, and all efforts should have teen input. In today's world, teens' own perspectives need to be heard and need to infuse all advocacy initiatives. As noted by one author, "nothing about us, without us."

• HCPs need to acquaint themselves with the unique characteristics of adolescence and how the teen years may be changing in the current society. Although we were all teens once, times have changed. We need to stay current to establish rapport with teens, relate to their needs and interests, and provide the best care possible!

• Although teens are sometimes embraced as a homogeneous group, the uniqueness and individuality of each teen must be considered. Realization that the perspectives of teens are as numerous as teens themselves ensures that although commonalities may exist, teens are unique and individually important!

SUGGESTED READING

Amieva, S., & Ferguson, S. (2011). Moving forward: Nurses are key to achieving the United Nations Development Program's millennium development goals. *International Nursing Review, 59*(1), 55–58.

Berlan, E. D., & Bravender, T. (2009). Confidentiality, consent, and caring for the adolescent patient. *Current Opinions in Pediatrics, 21*, 450–456.

Butts, J. B. (2005). Adolescent nursing ethics. In J. B. Butts & K. Rich, *Nursing ethics: Across the curriculum and into practice* (pp. 119–145). Boston, MA: Jones & Bartlett.

English, A., & Ford, C. (2004). The HIPAA privacy rule and adolescent: Legal questions and clinical challenges. *Perspectives on Sexual and Reproductive Health, 36*(2), 80–86.

Herrman, J. (2005). The teen brain as a work in progress: Implications for pediatric nurses. *Pediatric Nursing, 31*, 144–148.

Herrman, J. W. (2011). Teens and ethics: Development and decision-making. *DNA Reporter, 36*(2), 8.

Hester, C. J. (2004). Adolescent consent: Choosing the right path. *Issues in Comprehensive Pediatric Nursing, 27*, 27–37.

Lind, C., Anderson, B., & Oberle, K. (2003). Ethical issues in adolescent consent for research. *Nursing Ethics, 10*, 504–511.

Maradiegue, A. (2002). The Health Insurance Portability and Accountability Act and adolescents. *Pediatric Nursing, 28*(4), 417–420.

McNeely, C., & Blanchard, J. (2009). *The teen years explained: A guide to healthy adolescent development.* Baltimore, MD: Johns Hopkins Bloomburg School of Public Health.

Ott, M. A., Rosenberg, J. G., McBride, K. R., & Woodcox, S. G. (2011). How do adolescents view health? Implications for state health policy. *Journal of Adolescent Health, 48,* 398–403.

Roberson, A. J. (2007). Adolescent informed consent: Ethics, law, and theory to guide policy and nursing research. *Journal of Nursing Law, 11,* 191–196.

Serafini, T., Rye, B. J., & Drysdale, M. (Eds.). (2013). *Taking sides: Clashing views on adolescence.* New York, NY: McGraw-Hill.

Steinberg, L. (2008). *Adolescence.* New York, NY: McGraw-Hill.

Tillet, J. (2005). Adolescents and informed consent: Ethical and legal issues. *Journal of Perinatal and Neonatal Nursing, 19,* 112–121.

SUGGESTED WEBSITES

Education.com, Incorporated
www.education.com

The National Campaign to Prevent Teen and Unplanned Pregnancy
www.nationalcampaign.org

Advocates for Youth
www.advocatesforyouth.org

Kaiser Foundation
www.kff.org

The Innovation Center
www.theinnovationcenter.org

Girl Scouts
www.girlscouts.org

CityMatch
www.citymatch.org

ChildTrends
www.childtrends.org

The Search Institute
www.search-institute.org

Centers for Disease Control and Prevention
www.cdc.gov/healthyyouth

The Youth Activism Project
www.youthactivism.org

The Urban Institute
www.urban.org

American Medical Association
www.ama-assn.org

Society for Adolescent Medicine and Health
www.adolescenthealth.org

Healthy People
www.healthypeople.gov

Johns Hopkins School of Public Health
www.jhsph.edu

The World Health Organization
www.who.int/topics/adolescent_health

Wyman Center
www.wymancenter.org

Recommended Reading

Brizendine, L. (2006). *The female brain*. New York, NY: Morgan Road Books.

Carlson, D. (2004). *The teen brain book: Who and what are you?* Madison, CT: Bick.

Carter, R. (2009). *The human brain book*. New York, NY: DK.

Clavier, R. (2009). *Teen brain teen mind: What parents need to know to survive the adolescent years*. Ontario, Canada: Key Porter.

Covey, S. (1998). *The 7 habits of highly effective teens*. New York, NY: Simon and Schuster.

DiClemente, R. J., Santelli, J. S., & Crosby, R. A. (Eds.). (2009). *Adolescent health: Understanding and preventing risk behaviors*. San Francisco, CA: Jossey-Bass.

Family Planning Council. (2008). *Puberty's wild ride*. Philadelphia, PA: Author.

Feinstein, S. (2004). *Secrets of the teenage brain*. Thousand Oaks, CA: Corwin Press.

Feinstein, S. (2007). *Teaching the at-risk teenage brain*. Lanham, MD: Rowman & Littlefield.

Fenwick, E., & Smith, T. (1996). *Adolescence: A survival guide for parents and teenagers*. New York: DK.

Gibson, K. (2007). *Unlock the Einstein inside: Applying new brain science to wake the smart in your child*. Colorado Springs, CO: LearningRx.

Glazov, S. (2008). *What color is your brain?: A fun and fascinating approach to understanding yourself and others.* Thorofare, NJ: SLACK.

Henderson, A., & Champlin, S. (Eds.). (1998). *Promoting teen health: Linking schools, health organizations, and community.* Thousand Oaks, CA: Sage.

Kawashima, R. (2005). *Train your brain: 60 days to a better brain.* Teaneck, NJ: Kumon.

Levitin, D. J. (2006). *This is your brain on music: The science of a human obsession.* New York, NY: Plume.

McNeely, C., & Blanchard, J. (2009). *The teen years explained: A guide to healthy adolescent development.* Baltimore, MD: Johns Hopkins Bloomburg School of Public Health.

Mosee, S. W. (2009). *Professor, may I bring my baby to class? A student-mother's guide to college.* Philadelphia, PA: FCS Books.

Ponton, L. E. (1997). *The romance of risk: Why teenagers do the things they do.* New York, NY: Basic Books.

Romer, D. (Ed.). (2003). *Reducing the risk: Toward an integrated approach.* Thousand Oaks, CA: Sage.

Schalet, A. T. (2011). *Not under my roof: Parents, teens and the culture of sex.* Chicago, IL: University of Chicago Press.

Serafini, T., Rye, B. J., & Drysdale, M. (Eds.). (2013). *Taking sides: Clashing views on adolescence.* New York, NY: McGraw-Hill.

Sichel, D., & Driscoll, J. W. (2000). *Women's moods: What every woman must know about hormones, the brain, and emotional health.* New York, NY: Quill.

Steinberg, L. (2008). *Adolescence.* New York, NY: McGraw-Hill.

Stepp, L. S. (2007). *Unhooked: How young women pursue sex, delay love, and lose at both.* New York, NY: Riverhead Books.

Strauch, B. (2003). *The primal teen: What new discoveries about the teenage brain tell us about our kids.* New York, NY: Anchor.

Sweeney, M. S. (2009). *Brain: The complete mind, how it develops, how it works, and how to keep it sharp.* Washington, DC: National Geographic.

Walsh, D. (2004). *Why do they act that way? A survival guide to the adolescent brain for you and your teen.* New York, NY: Free Press.

Weinberger, D. R., Elevag, B., & Giedd, J. N. (2005). *The teen brain: A work in progress.* Washington, DC: The National Campaign to Prevent Teen and Unplanned Pregnancy.

Wright, T. D., & Richardson, J. W. (Eds.). (2012). *School-based health care: Advancing educational success and public health.* Washington, DC: American Public Health Association.

Index